The Ultimate Guide to Gut Health Reset for Women

Scientific Approach for A Leaky Gut with Holistic Nutrition to Vibrant Life, Weight Loss, and Hormonal Balance and Relieve Anxiety

Donna Johnson

Copyright 2024-

Donna Johnson

ISBN

Printed in the United States of America

Disclaimer

This publication is designed to provide competent and reliable information regarding the subject covered However, the views expressed in this publication are those of the author alone and should not be taken as expert instruction or professional advice The reader is responsible for his or her actions The author hereby disclaims any responsibility or liability whatsoever that is incurred from the use or application of the contents of this publication by the purchaser of the reader. The purchaser or reader is hereby responsible for his or her actions.

Table of Contents

Introduction...6

1. Understanding Gut Health....................................10

    The Gut: An Overview...10

    Importance of Gut Health in Women....................12

    The Gut-Brain Connection..................................14

    Microbiome Diversity and Its Impact...................16

2: Factors Affecting Women's Gut Health.................18

    Hormonal Changes and Gut Health.....................18

    Stress and Its Impact on the Gut........................20

    Diet and Nutrition..21

    Physical Activity and Gut Motility.......................24

3: Common Gut Health Issues in Women..................27

    Irritable Bowel Syndrome (IBS)..........................27

    Inflammatory Bowel Diseases............................29

    Leaky Gut Syndrome...31

    Bloating and Digestive Discomfort......................34

4: The Role of Diet in Gut Health.............................37

    Probiotics and Prebiotics...................................37

    Fiber-Rich Foods...39

    Elimination Diets...41

    Hydration and Gut Health..................................43

5: Mind-Gut Connection..46

    Stress Management Techniques..........................46

    Mindful Eating...48

    Yoga and Meditation for Gut Health...................50

    The Role of Sleep in Gut Health.........................52

6: Detoxification and Gut Health..............................54

Understanding Detoxification 54

Natural Detox Foods..56

Safe Detox Practices 58

Detox Myths Debunked...60

7: Gut Health through the Lifespan...63

Gut Health in Adolescence 63

Pregnancy and Gut Health 65

Menopause and Microbiome Changes 67

Aging and Gut Health 69

8: Functional Foods and Supplements 72

Choosing the Right Probiotics..72

Prebiotic Supplements 74

Vitamins and Minerals for Gut Health 76

Herbal Remedies for Digestive Health...78

9: Gut Health and Weight Management 81

Gut Microbiome and Obesity...81

Dieting and Gut Health...83

Exercise and Metabolic Health 85

10: Building a Gut-Healthy Lifestyle 87

Creating a Balanced Diet Plan...87

Integrating Physical Activity...89

Stress Reduction Techniques 91

Long-Term Gut Health Strategies..93

11: Overcoming Challenges in Gut Health...96

Dealing with Food Sensitivities 96

Navigating Dining Out...98

Emotional Eating and Gut Health 100

Staying Motivated and Consistent...102

12: Recipes for a Healthy Gut 105

Breakfast Ideas... 105

Lunch and Dinner Recipes 108

Snacks and Gut-Friendly Treats 112

Drinks and Smoothies 114

Introduction

The gut is a key player in the complex dance of health and wellbeing, with significant impact on our mental, emotional, and physical health. Women's bodies navigate distinct biological terrains characterized by fluctuating hormones, menstrual cycles, and varied life phases; thus, maintaining gut health becomes an essential component of overall well-being. Welcome to the Complete stomach Health Reset Guide for Women, a life-changing resource that explores the complex ecology of the stomach and provides women with a road map for regaining resilience, balance, and energy from the inside out.

The gut, a busy city teeming with billions of microbial residents collectively known as the gut microbiota, stands as a wonder of intricacy amid the maze that is the human body. Rather than only being observers, these little partners masterfully coordinate a symphony of immunological responses, metabolic processes, and neurotransmitter synthesis, influencing every aspect of our well-being. Our gut bacteria play a quiet role in regulating our emotions, immune system, and digestion. They also play a role in digestion and nutritional absorption.

For women, the relationship between hormone balance and intestinal health becomes a central theme that drives vitality. Women have a wide range of hormonal changes over their lives, from puberty to menopause. These changes have an impact on the microbial composition, intestinal permeability, and immune system across the gut environment. The gut acts as a guardian and a haven throughout periods of fluctuating estrogen, waxing and waning menstrual cycles, and the body's remarkable transformation during pregnancy and menopause. It is a gauge of internal balance and a storehouse of resistance.

However, in the hectic pace of contemporary life, the fragile balance of the stomach often gives way to the assault of poor food choices, ongoing stress, pollutants from the environment, and careless drug use. Environmental toxins that assault our bodies, processed foods loaded with sugar and artificial additives, long-term stressors that take over the nervous system, and antibiotics that indiscriminately destroy microbial communities all work together to upset the balance of the gut ecology, leading to dysbiosis, inflammation, and metabolic disorders.

The effects extend far beyond the boundaries of the digestive system and take the form of a variety of illnesses that affect the body, mind, and soul. The consequences of gut dysfunction throw a long, dark shadow over women's health, ranging from digestive issues like bloating, gas, and irritable bowel syndrome to systemic ailments including autoimmune illnesses, mental disorders, and metabolic syndrome. Fatigue depletes energy, mental fog impairs judgment, mood fluctuations upset emotional homeostasis, and hormone abnormalities undermine reproductive health eroding the fundamental foundation of femininity.

The Ultimate Guide to Gut Health Reset for Women heralds a paradigm change in the current paradigm of symptom suppression and fast fixes an invitation to go beyond the outward signs of sickness and address the underlying issues that may be hiding. With its foundation in the age-old wisdom of holistic treatment and its knowledge bolstered by the latest scientific discoveries, this book provides women with a roadmap to help them navigate the maze of gut health and recover resilience, energy, and radiant well-being from within.

The approach to gut health primarily consists of two steps: nourishing the microbiological buddies that live in our stomach and eliminating harmful pollutants from our body. Women have the ability to alter the environment of their stomachs by starving pathogenic invaders of food and cultivating a symbiotic relationship with helpful bacteria. This is achieved via the alchemy of diet. The canvas of nutrition appears as a pallet of healing colors, from fiber-rich fruits and vegetables that support microbial variety to fermented foods brimming with probiotic warriors, providing women with the means to nurture a thriving garden inside.

The art of restoration, which involves the cleansing, repair, and renewal of the gut environment, is equally important. Women set out on a journey of rejuvenation with specific treatments like prebiotic fibers, digestive enzymes, and herbal therapies; they cleanse the body's temple, bolster its defenses, and cultivate an internal sanctuary of vitality. In addition, mindful behaviors like stress reduction, good sleep hygiene, and mindful eating become recognized as holy routines that support women in the self-care sanctuary and nurture their body, mind, and soul.

However, the path to gut health extends beyond the boundaries of personal recovery, calling on women to foster a healthy culture that resonates across generations and communities. Women come together as stewards of health via the alchemy of compassionate action and shared knowledge. They advocate for food sovereignty, environmental stewardship, and regenerative agriculture, and they reclaim their birthright to robust health and vitality.

Let us take to heart Hippocrates' old wisdom as we set out on this life-changing journey: "All disease begins in the gut." The secret to solving the riddles of health and vitality is found in the maze-like gut, among the thriving microcosm of microbial life. This holy door invites women to reclaim their innate right to radiant well-being. I hope this book will be a lighthouse, a compass to help you find your way through the unknown seas of gut health and a reminder of the inherent ability that every woman has to change, heal, and flourish.

Here, in the Ultimate Guide to Gut Health Reset for Women, the path to vigor starts on the inside.

1. Understanding Gut Health

The Gut: An Overview

The gastrointestinal (GI) tract, often referred to as the gut, is a sophisticated system that is essential to our general health. It starts in the mouth and goes through the stomach, esophagus, small and large intestines, and finishes at the rectum.

Mouth and Esophagus: The mouth is where food is mechanically and chemically broken down to start the digestive process. The meal is subsequently transported to the stomach via the esophagus.

Stomach: Food is combined with digestive secretions in this area and transformed into chyme, a semi-liquid substance.

Small Intestine: The small intestine is where most nutrition absorption takes place. Villi and microvilli lining it increase the surface area available for absorption.

Large Intestine: It forms and stores excrement for excretion while absorbing water and electrolytes.

The microbiome, which is made up of billions of bacteria, viruses, and fungi, is found in the digestive tract. This microbiological community plays a key role in:

- Various foods' digestion
- Generating vital nutrients, such as vitamins B and K
- Defending against infections
- Controlling the immune system

The gut-brain axis is a network of communication that runs both ways between the gut and the brain. It is essential to:

- Mental and emotional well-being
- Stress reaction
- Control of appetite
- Dietary Influence on Gut Health

The gut microbiota is greatly influenced by the makeup of our food. Among the factors are:

1. Consumption of Fiber: Foods high in fiber encourage the development of good bacteria.
2. Probiotics and Prebiotics: A balanced microbiome is supported by probiotics, which are live beneficial bacteria, and prebiotics, which are food for these bacteria.
3. Prepared Foods: An imbalance in gut microbiota known as dysbiosis may result from excessive eating.

Numerous illnesses, including the following, may be attributed to an unhealthy gut:

- Digestive illnesses such as IBD and IBS
- Illnesses triggered by antibodies
- Metabolic conditions such as type 2 diabetes and obesity

Mental health issues include sadness and anxiety

It is essential to identify a sick stomach in order to take prompt action. Among the symptoms are:

- Digestive problems, such as gas, bloating, diarrhea, and constipation
- Inadvertent fluctuations in weight
- Weary
- Skin irritation

- Dietary intolerances

Importance of Gut Health in Women

Because of the complex interactions between hormones, the female lifecycle, and digestive health, gut health is particularly important for women. This section examines the relationship between gut health and a number of women's health-related factors, such as hormonal balance, mental health, and vulnerability to certain gut-related illnesses.

The Hormone-Gut Relationship

1   Menstrual Cycle: Variations in progesterone and estrogen levels may affect gut motility, which can lead to symptoms like constipation and bloating at various times of the cycle.
2   Pregnancy: Modifications in the gut microbiota during pregnancy may have an effect on immunological response and food absorption, as well as the health of the mother and fetus.
3   Menopause: Lower estrogen levels during menopause may have an impact on the microbiota and gut lining, which may increase gut permeability and cause digestive problems.

Reproductive and Gastrointestinal Health

1   Polycystic Ovary Syndrome (PCOS): New study indicates that gut dysbiosis and PCOS, a prevalent hormonal condition in women, are related.
2   Fertility: By influencing hormone control and lowering inflammation, a healthy gut microbiota may have an impact on fertility.

Digestive Health and the Brain-Gut Axis

1   Stress and Anxiety: Digestive problems associated with stress are more common in women. This is where the gut-brain axis comes in, since stress affects gut flora, which in turn affects mental health.

2   Mood Disorders: Research indicates that certain microbiome compositions are present in people with mood disorders, indicating a connection between gut health and conditions such as depression.

Women-Specific Intestinal Disorders

1   Irritable Bowel Syndrome (IBS): It is more common in women. Dietary variables, stress, and hormonal fluctuations are major influences.
2   Autoimmune Diseases: The frequency and symptoms of a few autoimmune diseases that affect the digestive system, such as Crohn's disease and ulcerative colitis, change depending on the gender.

Dietary and lifestyle factors' effects

1   Nutritional Requirements: Women have certain dietary requirements that affect gut health. For example, they need more iron and certain minerals that are absorbed by the stomach and promote bone growth.
2   Lifestyle Factors: Exercise, stress reduction, and good sleep are essential for preserving gut health, which has an impact on menstruation, pregnancy, and menopause.

Knowing how probiotics and prebiotics work to maintain gut health, especially in the case of bacterial vaginosis and IBS, is important.

Personalized nutrition refers to adjusting food choices to meet specific requirements for gut health while taking age, hormone levels, and pre-existing medical issues into account.

The Gut-Brain Connection

The enteric nervous system (ENS) in the stomach and the central nervous system (CNS) in the brain are connected in a bidirectional communication network known as the gut-brain axis.

Physiology and Anatomy of the Gut-Brain Axis

The ENS, sometimes known as the "second brain," is a system of reflexes and senses located in the gastrointestinal tract. It shares information with the brain via the vagus nerve.

The vagus nerve serves as the main pathway for both direction signal transmission between the brain and the intestines.

Neurotransmitters: A range of neurotransmitters, including gamma-aminobutyric acid (GABA) and serotonin, are produced by the stomach and are important for mood control.

Mental Health and Microbiome

1   Microbial Composition: The kinds of bacteria that reside in the stomach have the power to effect the synthesis of neurotransmitters and other substances that are involved in brain activity.
2   The phrase "microbiota-gut-brain axis" refers to the relationship between gut microbes and brain health, which may have an influence on behavior, mood, and cognitive abilities.

Mental Health and Digestive Health

1   Stress Response: The body's reaction to stress is influenced by the gut-brain axis. Prolonged stress may change gut flora, which might worsen symptoms associated with stress.

2   Mood Disorders: Alterations in gut microbiota have been connected to conditions including anxiety and depression. The possibility that altering gut flora might help certain ailments is being investigated.

3   Remembering and Cognition: New research points to a link between gut health and mental abilities, such as decision-making and remembering.

Dietary Influence on the Gut-Brain Axis

1   Probiotics and Mental Health: By affecting the gut-brain axis, certain probiotics, sometimes referred to as psychobiotics, may benefit mental health.

2   Food Routines: Eat a diet high in fruits, vegetables, whole grains, and lean meats to support brain health by fostering a healthy gut microbiota.

The Brain-Gut Axis and Neurological Conditions

1   Neuroinflammation: Prolonged intestinal inflammation may cause inflammation in the brain, which may be a factor in neurological conditions.

2   Neurodegenerative Diseases: Studies are examining the connections between disorders of the stomach and conditions such as Parkinson's and Alzheimer's.

Medicinal Strategies

1   Dietary and lifestyle modifications that promote gut health have been shown to have a significant impact on brain function.

2   Mind-Gut Therapies: The gut-brain axis may be positively impacted by strategies such as mindfulness exercises that focus on stress reduction and cognitive-behavioral therapy (CBT).

Microbiome Diversity and Its Impact

A diverse collection of bacteria living in our digestive system, the human gut microbiome is essential to our general health.

Meaning and Structure: Trillions of bacteria, viruses, fungi, and other microorganisms that inhabit the digestive system make up the gut microbiome.

Functions of the Microbiota these microbes are necessary for immunological system regulation, food digestion, vitamin synthesis, and bacterial defense.

The Value of Diversity in the Microbiome

1. Diversity and Health: Increased health is associated with a more varied gut microbiota. It strengthens the microbiome's resistance to diseases and helps it adjust to changes in the environment.
2. Variables Affecting Diversity: The diversity of the gut microbiome is influenced by a number of factors, including age, genetics, lifestyle, diet, and environmental exposures.

Health Effects of Microbiome Diversity

1. Digestive Health: Constipation, IBS, and IBD may all be avoided or treated with the help of a varied microbiome, which also promotes effective digestion.
2. Immune Function: It lowers the risk of allergies, autoimmune illnesses, and infections by helping to build and maintain a strong immune system.
3. Metabolic Health: Type 2 diabetes, obesity, and metabolic syndrome are all influenced by the close relationship between the variety of microbiomes and metabolic processes.

4   Mental Health: New studies point to a connection between gut microbiota and brain health, which may influence mental health disorders including anxiety and depression (the gut-brain axis).

Promoting the diversity of microbiomes

1   Diet: Eating a varied diet full of healthy grains, fruits, vegetables, fiber, and fermented foods encourages the growth of a diverse gut microbiota.

2   Probiotics and Prebiotics: To enhance microbiome diversity, include foods and supplements that include probiotics, which are live beneficial bacteria, and prebiotics, which are fibers that nourish helpful bacteria.

3   Lifestyle Factors: Keeping a healthy and varied microbiome also involves managing stress, getting enough sleep, and engaging in regular physical exercise.

Obstacles to the Diversity of Microbiomes

1   Medication and Antibiotics: Antibiotics may disturb the microbiota, even if they are sometimes important. Restoring gut health after antibiotic therapy and using them sparingly are crucial.

2   Contemporary Lifestyle: Microbiome diversity may be adversely affected by elements such as stress, sleep deprivation, and a high-sugar diet.

Gut Microbiome Testing: Scientific developments have made it feasible to examine the gut microbiomes of specific individuals, providing information about their own health and strategies for enhancing it.

Hormonal Changes and Gut Health

An inherent aspect of a woman's life cycle, hormonal swings affect several body systems, including her digestive system.

Periods and Digestive Health

Hormonal Fluctuations: Changes in progesterone and estrogen throughout the menstrual cycle might have an impact on gastrointestinal motility and cause symptoms like diarrhea, constipation, or bloating.

Symptoms of PMS and Digestion: These hormonal changes might cause stomach problems as part of premenstrual syndrome (PMS).

The Gut and Pregnancy

Hormonal Adaptations: Progesterone in especially during pregnancy may slow down digestion, which can result in typical problems like acid reflux and constipation.

Changes in the Microbiome: During pregnancy, the mother's changing body and the fetal health are thought to be supported by changes in the gut microbiota.

Nutritional Needs: Pregnancy-related increases in nutritional requirements may have an impact on gut health and call for dietary modifications.

Gut Health and Menopause

Estrogen Decline: The menopause, which is characterized by a decrease in estrogen, may have an impact on gut motility and raise the possibility of gastrointestinal issues.

Increased Risk of Gut Disorders: Women who have gone through menopause may be more susceptible to illnesses like GERD and irritable bowel syndrome (IBS).

Hormones of the Thyroid and Gut Health

Hypothyroidism: Disorders such as hypothyroidism may cause constipation by slowing down the motility of the intestines.

Hyperthyroidism: On the other hand, hyperthyroidism may accelerate the motility of the stomach, which may result in diarrhea and other digestive problems.

Gut and Stress Hormones

Cortisol: Stress causes the production of cortisol, which may have an adverse effect on gut health by increasing permeability and changing gut motility. This may result in conditions such as leaky gut syndrome.

Contraceptives with hormones and gut health

Birth Control Pills: Although research in this field is still in its early stages, hormonal contraceptives have the potential to alter gut flora and gut health.

The Gut and Hormone Replacement Therapy (HRT)

HRT has the ability to change the makeup of the gut microbiota, which may have an impact on gut health.

Hormone Balancing: Gut problems associated with menopause might be lessened with properly administered HRT.

Merely focusing on a well-balanced diet that includes enough of fiber, probiotics, and water will help lessen the negative effects of hormones on the gastrointestinal tract.

Exercise: Getting regular exercise helps enhance gut motility and gut health in general.

Stress and Its Impact on the Gut

Stress, a ubiquitous occurrence in contemporary life, significantly affects gut health, especially in women.

The Body's reaction to Stress: When the body experiences stress, chemicals like cortisol and adrenaline are released as part of the fight-or-flight reaction. The digestive system may be affected by this reaction.

Stress: Acute stress may result in short-term pain related to the digestive system, whilst persistent stress can create long-term problems related to the digestive system.

Modified Digestion: Stress has the ability to increase or decrease gut motility, which may result in symptoms such as cramping in the stomach, diarrhea, or constipation.

Gut Sensitivity: Stress, particularly in diseases like irritable bowel syndrome (IBS), may enhance gut sensitivity and amplify the sensation of pain and discomfort.

Microbial Imbalance: Stress may throw off the delicate balance of gut flora, resulting in dysbiosis and subsequent damage to the gut's general health.

Impact on immunological Function: Stress-induced alterations in the microbiome may impact immunological responses since the gut contains a significant portion of the immune system.

Women's Stress-Related Gut Disorders

Greater Frequency of IBS: IBS is more common in women, and stress is a well-known initiator of IBS symptoms.

Stress may make symptoms of gastroesophageal reflux disease (GERD) worse by causing the creation of more stomach acid.

Gut Health and Psychological Stress

Mental Health and the Gut: Anxiety and depression are two conditions that may exacerbate gut health, which can lead to a vicious cycle in which poor gut health exacerbates mental health issues.

Eating Behaviors: Stress may cause changes in eating habits that can affect gut health by either suppressing appetite or causing overeating.

Women's Hormonal Fluctuations: Stress may exacerbate problems with gut health by interacting with hormonal changes that occur during menstruation, pregnancy, or menopause.

Techniques to Treat Gut Problems Caused by Stress

1   Mind-Gut Connection: Stress management and gut health may be enhanced by practices such as yoga, meditation, and mindfulness.

2   Frequent Exercise: Studies have shown that exercise may lower stress, enhance gastrointestinal motility, and enhance general health.

3   Diet and Nutrition: During times of stress, eating a well-balanced diet high in fiber, probiotics, and minerals will help maintain gut health.

4   Sufficient Sleep: Restorative sleep is essential for gut health and stress management.

Diet and Nutrition

Nutrition and diet are essential for preserving women's intestinal health.

Balanced Diet: For intestinal health, a diet high in a variety of nutrients is essential. A variety of fruits, vegetables, nutritious grains, lean meats, and healthy fats are included in this.

Consumption of Fiber: Whole grains, legumes, fruits, vegetables, and other foods high in fiber are necessary for a healthy digestive system and regular bowel motions.

Hydration: Drinking enough water promotes healthy digestion by facilitating the production of stool and the absorption of nutrients.

Particular Nutrients' Effects on Gut Health

Probiotics are live, helpful bacteria that are present in fermented foods such as kefir, sauerkraut, and yogurt. They aid in the maintenance of a healthy gut microbiota.

Prebiotics: Found in foods like onions, garlic, and asparagus, prebiotics nourish and maintain a healthy gut flora.

Antioxidants: Consuming foods high in antioxidants might boost immunity and lessen gastrointestinal inflammation.

Specifically Needed Nutrition for Women

Iron: Women often need extra iron due to monthly blood loss. Iron is essential for general health and might have an influence on gut health.

Calcium and vitamin D: These elements may be effectively absorbed in the event of a healthy stomach and are essential for bone health, particularly in postmenopausal women.

Nutritional Factors in All Life Stages

Menstruation: Iron and vitamin-rich diets may help offset the loss of blood that occurs with menstruation.

Pregnancy and Lactation: During pregnancy and lactation, the body need more nutrients. Particularly significant are fiber, iron, calcium, and folate.

Menopause: In order to preserve gut health and avoid weight gain, postmenopausal women may need to modify their diet.

Typical Dietary Mistakes

1   Processed Foods: Consuming a lot of processed food might upset the gut flora and cause digestive problems.
2   Diets high in sugar and fat have the potential to change gut flora, which may lead to inflammation and digestive issues.
3   Food Sensitivities: A customized diet is necessary to manage food sensitivities such as gluten, dairy, and others that may affect gut health.

Diet's Function in Conditions Related to the Gut

Irritable Bowel Syndrome (IBS): The low-FODMAPS diet is one diet that may help control IBS symptoms.

The kind and severity of Inflammatory Bowel Disease (IBD) may influence different nutritional regimens.

Adopting a Diet That Is Gut-Healthy

Meal planning: Putting together nutritious meals with foods that are good for the stomach.

Eating mindfully involves observing the effects that various meals have on your body and modifying your diet appropriately.

Physical Activity and Gut Motility

Especially for women, physical exercise has a crucial but often disregarded role in supporting intestinal health.

The Relationship between Gut Health and Exercise

Increasing Gut Motility: It has been shown that regular exercise increases gut motility, which facilitates more effective digestion and lowers the incidence of constipation.

Modulation of the Gut Microbiome: Physical activity has a beneficial impact on the composition and variety of the gut microbiota, leading to a more robust gut environment.

Exercise and Intestinal Disorders

Exercise has been shown to help women with Irritable Bowel Syndrome (IBS) symptoms, such as bloating and stomach discomfort.

Inflammatory Bowel Disease (IBD): Moderate exercise may help people with IBD feel better overall and enhance their quality of life, even if moderate exercise can sometimes make symptoms worse.

The Effects of Exercise and Hormones on Gut Health

Menstrual Cycle: Exercise might lessen the effects of digestive problems associated with the menstrual cycle, such as bloating and constipation.

Menopause: Regular exercise helps offset the effects of menopause, such as reduced metabolism and decreased motility of the stomach, on gut health.

Kinds of Physical Activities That Are Beneficial

Aerobic Exercises: Exercises that increase intestinal activity and enhance gut health include running, cycling, swimming, and brisk walking.

Strength Training: Gaining muscular mass helps enhance metabolic well-being, which in turn promotes intestinal health.

Pilates and yoga: By putting the body in certain positions, these exercises may directly stimulate the digestive organs and lower stress, both of which have a detrimental effect on gut health.

Exercise's Function in Stress Reduction

Lowering Cortisol Levels: Engaging in regular physical exercise can reduce stress hormone levels, which may have a favorable effect on gut health.

Mind-Body Connection: Mind-gut integration may be reinforced by exercise practices such as yoga and tai chi, which can improve digestion and overall wellbeing.

Customizing Workout Plans to Meet Specific Needs

Personalized Exercise Plans: When selecting an exercise program, women should take into account many criteria such as age, fitness level, and pre-existing medical disorders.

Consistency and Moderation: Intermittent, high-intensity exercises are not as good for gut health as regular, moderate activity.

Obstacles and Things to Think About

Overtraining: Getting too much exercise might cause intestinal problems including "leaky gut" (increased intestinal permeability).

Nutrition and Hydration: In order to preserve gut health and restore depleted nutrients, it is crucial to consume the right foods and beverages, particularly after physical activity.

3: Common Gut Health Issues in Women

Irritable Bowel Syndrome (IBS)

Definition: A range of symptoms, such as bloating, constipation, diarrhea, or both, and stomach discomfort, are indicative of irritable bowel syndrome (IBS).

Prevalence in Women: Compared to Men, women are more prone to experience distinct stress reactions and hormonal fluctuations that may contribute to the development of IBS.

Signs and Prognosis

Constipation, diarrhea, gas, bloating, cramps, and/or chronic stomach discomfort are typical symptoms.

Diagnostic standards: Patterns of symptoms and ruling out other illnesses are usually used to make a diagnosis. The Rome IV standards are often used.

Reasons and Initiators

Gut-Brain Axis: A major contributing factor to IBS is the interaction between the gut and the brain. Symptoms may worsen as a result of psychological issues and stress.

Hormonal Fluctuations: The symptoms of IBS might be influenced by the menstrual cycle, pregnancy, and menopause.

Dietary factors: A number of foods and drinks, such as those rich in fructooligosaccharides (FODMAPS), gluten, dairy, caffeine, and alcohol, might intensify symptoms.

Microbiome Imbalance: IBS has been connected to dysbiosis, or an imbalance in gut flora.

Women-Specific Factors to Consider in IBS

Impact on Menstrual Cycle: A lot of women say that their IBS symptoms are worse either before or right after their periods.

IBS and pregnancy: Changes in pregnancy may impact the symptoms of IBS, often necessitating modifications to treatment plans.

Menopause and IBS: The hormonal shifts that occur at this time might impact IBS symptoms, often requiring an alternative treatment plan.

Handling and Medical Interventions

Dietary Adjustments: It might be helpful to identify specific dietary triggers, increase fiber intake, and adopt a low-FODMAP diet.

Stress Management: There are strategies to assist control the stress-related aspect of IBS, including mindfulness, cognitive-behavioral therapy (CBT), and relaxation exercises.

Medication: Antispasmodics, laxatives, and antidiarrheals are a few examples of drugs that may be recommended based on symptoms. Probiotics may also be advantageous.

Physical Activity: Consistent exercise helps lower stress and improve bowel movements.

Changes in Lifestyle

Mindful Eating: You may lessen the symptoms of IBS by being aware of your eating habits and steering clear of heavy meals.

Hydration: Drinking enough water is crucial, particularly for IBS patients who have constipation often.

Rest and Sleep: Getting enough good-quality sleep may help control the symptoms of IBS.

Getting Expert Assistance

Consultation with a gastroenterologist: For diagnosis and treatment, particularly in extreme circumstances.

Dietitian Advice: For individualized dietary recommendations and the use of the low-FODMAPS diet.

Support for Mental Health: For managing stress, anxiety, or depression that might be associated with IBS.

Inflammatory Bowel Diseases

The term "inflammatory bowel diseases" (IBD) refers to a group of chronic inflammatory gastrointestinal disorders that include Crohn's disease and ulcerative colitis.

Inflammatory Bowel Diseases Are:

The hallmark of Crohn's disease is inflammation, which may develop anywhere in the digestive system and often affects the two deeper layers of the intestinal wall.

The lining of the large intestine (colon) and the rectum are the main sites of inflammation and ulceration in ulcerative colitis.

Female Epidemiology: Due to hormonal and reproductive reasons, women with IBD may face particular symptoms and difficulties.

Signs and Prognosis

Frequent symptoms include exhaustion, weight loss, rectal bleeding, stomach discomfort, and chronic diarrhea. Infertility problems and irregular menstruation are other possible experiences for women.

Tools for Diagnosis: A combination of endoscopic procedures, imaging investigations, and laboratory testing, including as colonoscopies, MRIs, and blood tests, are often used to make a diagnosis.

Reasons and Danger Elements

Genetic Predisposition: The risk is increased if there is a family history of IBD.

Environmental Triggers: Stress, diet, and lifestyle are considered to be important factors.

Immune System Dysfunction: An aberrant immune response to the flora in the gut is a component of IBD.

IBD in Women: Particular Issues

Impact on Menstrual Cycle: Women with IBD may have more painful and irregular menstrual cycles.

IBD and pregnancy: IBD may affect a woman's ability to conceive, the course of her pregnancy, and the medications she takes.

Menopause and IBD: Changes in hormones at this time might impact the symptoms of IBD and how well a treatment plan works.

Dietary considerations

Risks associated with malnutrition: It's important to keep a sufficient diet because of malabsorption or decreased appetite.

Dietary Management: Customized diets may support nutritional balance and aid in symptom management. Refusing to eat trigger foods is often advised.

Medication: A variety of pharmaceuticals, such as biologics, immunosuppressants, and anti-inflammatory drugs, are used to treat inflammatory bowel disease (IBD).

Surgical Interventions: To remove damaged GI tract segments, surgery can be required in extreme situations.

Way of Life and Complementary Medicine

Stress Management: Since stress may worsen the symptoms of IBD, it's important to learn stress-reduction strategies.

Exercise: Getting regular exercise may help control symptoms and enhance general health.

Alternative Therapies: Herbal medicines, probiotics, and acupuncture have helped some individuals find relief; however, you should speak with a healthcare professional before using any of them.

A Look at Women's Health

Fertility and Family Planning: Since IBD might impact fertility, it's critical to have family planning conversations.

Bone Health: Osteoporosis is more common in postmenopausal women and may be exacerbated by long-term IBD and certain therapies.

Leaky Gut Syndrome
Increased intestinal permeability, sometimes referred to as leaky gut syndrome, is a disorder in which the small intestine's lining is harmed, enabling germs, toxic waste products, and undigested food particles to "leak" into the bloodstream.

Comprehending Leaky Gut Syndrome

Conceptual Overview: Leaky Gut Syndrome is defined by a weakening of the intestinal barrier, which allows chemicals that are ordinarily prohibited from entering the circulation to slip through.

Symptoms: These might include eczema, persistent diarrhea, bloating, constipation, exhaustion, and nutritional deficits.

Reasons and Involving Elements

Diet: A diet heavy in carbohydrates, processed foods, and alcohol may be a factor in the development of leaky gut.

Medication: Some pharmaceuticals, such antibiotics and nonsteroidal anti-inflammatory drugs (NSAIDs), may harm the intestinal lining and disturb the balance of gut flora.

Prolonged Stress: Prolonged stress has the potential to impair immunity and exacerbate gastrointestinal inflammation.

Toxins: The stomach may become inflamed when exposed to environmental toxins.

Leaky Gut and the Health of Women

Hormonal Fluctuations: Variations in the menstrual cycle, pregnancy, and menopause might worsen symptoms by altering the permeability of the gut.

Autoimmune Diseases: Leaky gut may contribute to the development of autoimmune disorders, which are more common in women.

Identification and Evaluation

Difficulties in Diagnosing: Leaky gut syndrome is difficult to diagnose since there is no approved test for it.

Evaluation of symptoms, dietary analysis, and specialized testing (such as zonulin levels or intestinal permeability tests) are some of the methods used by healthcare professionals in the assessment process.

Dietary control

Anti-inflammatory Diet: Limiting inflammatory foods while focusing on a diet high in fiber, whole foods, and minerals might be helpful.

Probiotics and prebiotics may enhance the function of the intestinal barrier by assisting in the restoration of a healthy gut flora.

Supplements: L-glutamine, zinc, and omega-3 fatty acids are a few examples of supplements that may aid with gut healing.

Modifications to Lifestyle

Stress reduction: You may lessen the negative effects of stress on your gut health by practicing yoga, meditation, and mindfulness.

Exercise: Regular, mild exercise helps enhance general health and gastrointestinal motility.

Sleep hygiene: Getting enough sleep is crucial for maintaining gut health and general wellbeing.

Complementary and Alternative Therapies

Herbal Remedies: Some herbs, such as marshmallow root and slippery elm, may aid in the repair of the digestive system.

Another strategy for treating symptoms and stress is acupuncture.

Health Care Procedures

Treating Underlying problems: It is essential to treat any underlying problems, like autoimmune diseases or IBS.

Medications: Specific leaky gut symptoms or problems may be treated with medications.

Bloating and Digestive Discomfort

Frequent gastrointestinal problems including bloating and digestive pain are more frequent in women because of a variety of physiological and lifestyle variables.

Recognizing Bloating and Discomfiting Digestive System

Definition and Symptoms: Bloating is the term for an abdomen-wide sensation of fullness or swelling that is often accompanied by symptoms like gas, discomfort, and abdominal pain.

Prevalence in Women: Women are more likely to have these symptoms than males are due in part to hormonal cycles, food choices, and stress levels.

Reasons for Digestive Discomfort and Bloating

Dietary factors: Bloating and increased gas production may result from consuming high-fiber meals, fizzy beverages, and specific carbs.

Hormonal Changes: Bloating may result from changes in gastrointestinal motility and fluid retention brought on by menstruation, pregnancy, and menopause.

Functional Gastrointestinal Disorders: Bloating and pain are common symptoms of conditions such as irritable bowel syndrome (IBS).

Lifestyle Factors: Stress, a sedentary lifestyle, and erratic eating patterns may all make these problems worse.

Effect on the Health of Women

Psychological Impact: Prolonged gas and discomfort may have a negative impact on mental health, which can result in tension and worry.

Quality of Life: Daily activities and general well-being may be negatively impacted by chronic digestive problems.

Diagnostic Method

Medical assessment: It is essential to do a comprehensive assessment in order to rule out underlying diseases such as celiac disease, IBS, or food intolerances.

Symptom Tracking: Maintaining a diet and symptom journal might assist in determining probable causes and trends.

Nutritional Control

Identifying Triggers: Steer clear of or restrict foods like beans, onions, and dairy items that are known to induce bloating.

Portion control: Eating more often and smaller meals may reduce gastrointestinal distress.

Consumption of Fiber: Over time, a gradual increase in dietary fiber may decrease bloating and enhance gastrointestinal motility.

Changes in Lifestyle

Frequent Exercise: Exercise helps decrease gas buildup and enhance intestinal motility.

Hydration: Drinking enough water, in particular, may help reduce bloating.

Stress management: Methods like yoga, mindfulness, and meditation may help with digestive problems brought on by stress.

Alternative and Medical Therapies

Over-the-Counter Remedies: Activated charcoal and simethicone are two items that help temporarily relieve gas and bloating.

Probiotics: These may enhance digestive health by balancing the intestinal flora.

Herbal Teas: The digestive properties of peppermint, ginger, and chamomile teas are well-known.

Preventive Actions

Mindful Eating: Eating slowly and properly chewing your meal might help with digestion and less air swallowing.

Steer clear of carbonated beverages since they may exacerbate bloating and gas.

Frequent Medical Exams: Regular exams may assist in detecting and treating any underlying medical conditions that may be impacting digestion.

4: The Role of Diet in Gut Health

Probiotics and Prebiotics

Overall health depends on the variety and balance of the gut microbiota, and this microbial ecology is greatly influenced by nutrition.

Knowing About Prebiotics and Probiotics

Probiotics are defined as live microorganisms, mostly yeast and bacteria that provide health advantages when ingested in sufficient quantities.

Prebiotics are defined as indigestible dietary ingredients, mainly fibers and oligosaccharides that encourage the development and activity of good gut flora.

Probiotic and prebiotic synergy: Prebiotics feed probiotics, which in turn improves gut health when they are combined.

Advantages of Probiotics for Health

Boosting Gut Flora: Probiotics support the maintenance of a balanced population of good gut bacteria.

Immune Function: They contribute to immune system modulation, which lowers the risk of infections and some autoimmune illnesses.

Digestive Health: Probiotics may help reduce the symptoms of constipation, diarrhea, and IBS, among other gastrointestinal illnesses.

Mental Health: New study indicates that gut health and mental health are related, and that probiotics may help with mental health issues including anxiety and sadness.

Sources of Probiotics

Fermented Foods: Probiotics are abundant in yogurt, kefir, sauerkraut, tempeh, and miso.

Pills: For those who struggle to include fermented foods in their diet, probiotic pills are available.

Advantages of Prebiotics for Health

Support for the Gut Microbiota: Prebiotics promote the development of Bifidobacteria and Lactobacilli, two types of helpful gut bacteria.

Digestive System: Prebiotics help enhance gut health and bowel regularity by fostering good bacteria.

Nutrient Absorption: They have the ability to improve the body's absorption of minerals that are crucial for healthy bones, such as magnesium and calcium.

Where to Get Prebiotics

Dietary Sources: Garlic, onions, leeks, asparagus, bananas, whole grains, and apples are foods rich in prebiotics.

Supplements: Supplements are available for people who need to enhance their consumption of prebiotics.

Supplementing the Diet with Probiotics and Prebiotics

Balanced Approach: A wide range of good bacteria may be guaranteed by include a variety of probiotic and prebiotic items in the diet.

Techniques for Cooking: Mastering the preparation and usage of fermented foods may improve their flavor and ability to be incorporated into meals.

Individual Tolerance: When introducing prebiotics and fermented foods into their diet, some persons may first feel bloated or gassy.

Thoughts and Cautions

Personal Health issues: Before taking probiotics or prebiotics, those with specific health issues, such as compromised immune systems, should speak with a healthcare provider.

Supplement Quality: It's important to choose reputable brands with tested strains and sufficient colony-forming units (CFUs) when picking supplements.

Fiber-Rich Foods

Dietary fiber is essential for preserving intestinal health. It helps with digestion, but it also affects blood sugar regulation, weight control, and cardiovascular health, among other areas of health.

Types and Definition: Dietary fiber is the portion of plant foods that cannot be digested. There are two primary kinds of fiber: insoluble fiber, which helps to thicken stool, and soluble fiber, which dissolves in water and is digested by gut bacteria.

Sources of fiber: Fruits, vegetables, whole grains, legumes, nuts, and seeds are examples of common sources.

Fiber's Health Benefits

Digestive Health: Fiber keeps the digestive system healthy and promotes regular bowel movements, which help avoid constipation.

Gut Microbiome: Eating meals high in fiber nourishes the good bacteria in the stomach, fostering a balanced gut flora.

Weight management: Foods high in fiber are more satisfying, which helps regulate hunger and promote weight management.

Blood Sugar Control: Soluble fiber contributes to blood sugar regulation by slowing down the absorption of sugar.

Lowering Bad Cholesterol: Some soluble fiber varieties may lower bad cholesterol levels, promoting heart health.

Suggested Daily Consumption

General Guidelines: Although the recommended daily intake of fiber varies, men and women should typically strive for roughly 38 grams and 25 grams of fiber, respectively, per day.

Including Fiber in Your Diet

Gradual Increase: It's important to make sure you're getting enough water and to gradually increase your fiber intake to prevent upset stomach.

Various Sources: Consuming a range of meals high in fiber guarantees a diversity of fibers and optimizes health benefits.

Supplements against Whole Foods: Although supplements have their place, whole foods provide more nutrients and are a better source of fiber.

Obstacles and Things to Think About

Individual Tolerance: When increasing their fiber intake, some persons may feel gas or bloating.

Certain Medical Conditions: People who suffer from certain digestive disorders, such Crohn's disease or IBS, may need to adjust how much fiber they consume and should speak with a doctor.

Preparing meals and cooking

Recipes High in Fiber: You may increase your intake of fiber by including whole grains, lentils, and a range of veggies in your meals.

Snack Ideas: Easy and high in fiber snacks include nuts, seeds, and fresh fruit.

Reading Food Labels: When shopping, knowing what to look for on food labels might help you choose high-fiber items.

Elimination Diets

A technique called an elimination diet is used to find foods that a person may be allergic to or that may be aggravating health problems, especially those connected to the stomach.

Definition and Goals: An elimination diet consists of taking certain foods or food categories out of the diet for a while, then gradually adding them back in to see whether there are any negative effects.

Application: Food intolerances, allergies, irritable bowel syndrome (IBS), and other autoimmune illnesses may all be identified with the use of these diets.

Typical Foods That Elimination Diets Target

Dairy Products: Digestion may be worse by lactose intolerance or sensitivity to dairy proteins.

Gluten: Gastrointestinal symptoms may arise from celiac disease or gluten intolerance.

Soy, nuts, and eggs are common allergies that might result in negative responses.

Processed foods: Often loaded with preservatives and additives that might irritate certain people's digestive systems.

Putting an End to an Elimination Diet

Phase of planning: Depending on symptoms and medical history, choose which foods to cut out by speaking with a dietician or healthcare professional.

Phase of Elimination: Usually takes two to six weeks, during which time any items that may be suspected are avoided.

Phase of Reintroduction: Reintroduce foods one at a time, gradually, while keeping an eye out for symptoms.

Observation and Record-Keeping

Food Diary: Identifying certain triggers requires keeping a thorough record of items eaten and any symptoms encountered.

Symptom tracking involves keeping track of how the food affects your general wellbeing, energy levels, and digestive complaints.

Difficulties and Hazards

Nutritional shortages: If particular food categories are eliminated over an extended period of time without proper management, nutritional shortages may result.

Effect on Lifestyle: Eating habits and meal planning may need to be drastically altered due to the diet's potential for restriction.

Assistance and direction

Professional Assistance: To properly carry out an elimination diet and analyze the findings, ongoing assistance from healthcare specialists is essential.

Nutritional Balance: Following a dietitian's advice to ensure a balanced intake of nutrients from supplements or other dietary sources.

Strategies after Dieting

Long-Term Dietary Modifications: Long-term dietary adjustments could be required in light of the elimination diet's results.

Handling Hypersensitivity: creating plans to prevent or reduce exposure to recognized triggers; examples include stating dietary requirements while dining out and reviewing labels.

Hydration and Gut Health

Staying hydrated is essential for preserving intestinal health. Sufficient consumption of fluids is crucial for several digestive procedures and may greatly influence the general functioning of the gastrointestinal tract.

Hydration's Significance for Digestive Health

Digestive Processes: Water is necessary for food to be properly digested. It helps the food break down in the stomach and makes it easier for the intestines to absorb nutrients.

Bowel Movements: Drinking enough water makes feces softer and keeps constipation, a frequent digestive problem, at bay.

Dehydration's Effects on Gut Health

Constipation: As the body absorbs more water from the colon, dehydration may cause firmer stool and constipation.

Digestive Discomfort: Bloating, cramping, and indigestion may be brought on by a low fluid intake.

Effect on Gut Microbiome: Prolonged dehydration may have a deleterious effect on the equilibrium of the gut microbiota.

Suggested Water Consumption

General Recommendations: Although personal requirements differ, it is generally advised to consume 8 to 10 glasses (or about 2 liters) of water daily. But requirements might change depending on things like weather, level of physical activity, and general health.

Hydration and Various Phases of Life

Pregnancy and lactation: During these times, women's bodies need more fluids to sustain the increasing needs.

Aging: Elderly people should take extra care to ensure they are getting enough fluids since they may have a decreased thirst sensation.

Sources of Hydration

The most efficient and direct source of hydration is water.

Other Fluids: You may increase your fluid intake by drinking herbal teas, broths, and certain meals that are high in hydration, such as fruits and vegetables.

Restricting Diuretics: Alcohol and caffeine-containing beverages should be used in moderation since they may have diuretic effects.

Keeping an eye on your hydration levels

Urine Color: Seeing the color of pee is an easy approach to keep an eye on your level of hydration. Dark pee implies dehydration, whereas pale yellow urine usually indicates enough hydration.

Thirst: Although it's a late warning sign of dehydration, thirst is nevertheless a crucial indication that shouldn't be disregarded.

Including Hydration in Everyday Activities

Frequent Water Breaks: Making it a habit to hydrate yourself with water throughout the day.

Hydration applications: Monitoring water consumption and creating reminders using smartphone applications.

Keeping a Water Bottle on Hand: It might motivate more frequent sips of water throughout the day to have a bottle close at hand.

Difficulties in Retaining Hydration

Individual Variability: Hydration requirements may be influenced by variables such as body size, exercise level, and ambient temperature.

Health Conditions: Customized fluid intake guidelines may be necessary for certain health concerns, such as renal or heart difficulties.

5: Mind-Gut Connection

Stress Management Techniques

The mind-gut connection is intricate and reciprocal; stress has a big influence on gut health and vice versa.

The phrase "gut-brain axis" describes the network of communication that includes the microbiota, enteric nervous system, and central nervous system that runs between the gut and the brain.

Stress's Effect on the Gut: Prolonged stress may change the balance of gut bacteria, increase gut permeability (causing leaky gut syndrome), and affect gut motility.

Strategies for Stress Reduction for Gut Health

Mindfulness Meditation: Stress may have a negative impact on gut health, but mindfulness meditation helps lessen it. It entails concentrating on and embracing the current situation without passing judgment.

Deep Breathing Exercises: By triggering the body's relaxation response, methods such as diaphragmatic breathing may lower stress and perhaps even enhance intestinal health.

Progressive muscle relaxation is a technique that helps reduce stress in both the body and mind. It entails tensing and then releasing various muscle groups.

Yoga and Tai Chi: These forms of exercise combine physical poses with breathing techniques and meditation to help lower stress and promote better gut health.

Therapy based on cognitive behavior (CBT)

Function in Stress Management: Cognitive Behavioral Therapy (CBT) may assist in addressing the cognitive processes that lead to stress, which may mitigate the symptoms of stress-related digestive problems.

Use: Cognitive behavioral therapy (CBT) methods include recognising and questioning harmful beliefs as well as creating constructive thought patterns and coping mechanisms.

Frequent Exercise

Exercise as a Stress Reliever: Engaging in regular physical exercise can dramatically lower stress levels, which may benefit gut health.

Exercise Types: Aerobic activities, like jogging, swimming, or walking, might be very beneficial.

Nutritional Aspects

A well-balanced diet that is high in natural foods and low in processed foods may help maintain gastrointestinal and mental health.

Keep Stimulants Away: cutting down on sugar and caffeine use, which may worsen stress and have a detrimental effect on gut health.

The Value of Getting Enough Sleep

Stress and Sleep: Insufficient sleep may lead to increased stress levels, which can impact intestinal health. Getting enough sleep is essential to keeping the mind-gut connection in balance.

Hygiene Practices for Sleep: Enhancing sleep quality may be achieved by establishing a regular sleep pattern, making your bedroom cozy, and reducing screen time before bed.

Activities for Relaxation and Social Support

Social Networks: Having a strong social network may assist with stress management and emotional support.

Hobbies and Activities that Encourage Relaxation: Reading, drawing, gardening, and other hobbies and activities that encourage relaxation may help lower stress levels.

Mindful Eating

The practice of mindful eating is focusing entirely on the eating experience, being aware of the signals your body gives you about when you're hungry and full, and appreciating the sensory qualities of food.

Definition and guiding principles: The goal of mindful eating is to fully attend to all feelings, urges, and bodily signals throughout the eating process.

As opposed to Mindless Eating: Ignoring the body's cues and the emotional connection to food, mindless eating often results in overeating and intestinal pain.

The Health Benefits of Mindful Eating for the Gut

Better Digestion: Mindful eating helps improve digestion and lessen pain by eating slowly and digesting food completely.

Controlling Appetite: It is better for gut health to avoid overeating and undereating by paying attention to hunger and fullness signals.

Stress Reduction: By transforming meals into a kind of meditation, mindful eating helps lessen stress and its detrimental effects on the digestive system.

Methods for Putting Mindful Eating Into Practice

Eating Distraction-Free: To ensure that you give your whole attention to your meal, turn off devices like TVs and cellphones.

Eating in reaction to physical hunger signals rather than emotional hunger is known as listening to hunger cues.

Chewing Carefully: Giving meals a good chewing experience improves digestion and nutritional absorption.

Taking note of the flavor, texture, and scent of food is a key component in appreciating it.

Conscious Eating in Everyday Life

Starting Small: Start with only one mindful meal each day and work your way up to a larger meal.

Mindful Meal Preparation: Cooking may be a more mindful experience when done with awareness and presence.

Mindful grocery shopping involves selecting foods with awareness of their nutritional value and the requirements of the body.

Overcoming Obstacles in Intentional Eating

Adapting mindful eating to a busy lifestyle may be achieved by practicing it at less stressful meals, for example.

Understanding and resolving the emotional components of eating behaviors is known as "emotional eating."

Particular Diets and Mindful Eating

Integration with nutritional Restrictions: Applying the concepts of mindful eating to particular diets, whether they be nutritional, ethical, or health-related.

Using mindful eating as a non-restrictive method of maintaining a healthy weight is known as mindful eating for weight management.

Yoga and Meditation for Gut Health

Ancient techniques like yoga and meditation have shown amazing advantages for mental and physical well-being, including digestive system health.

Yoga for Digestive Health

Mechanism of Action: Yoga incorporates meditation, deliberate breathing, and physical postures. Combining these two may help lower stress, which is one of the major things impacting gut health. Furthermore, some yoga postures may directly stimulate and massage the stomach organs, enhancing digestion and reducing bloating and constipation.

Positive Yoga Pose: Asanas (Knee-to-Chest Pose), Pavanamuktasana (Wind-Relieving Pose), and twisting postures are among the asanas that encourage intestinal motility and alleviate gas. It is advised to do Thunderbolt Pose, or Vajrasana, after eating to improve digestion.

The Vagus Nerve and Yoga: Regular yoga practice may improve gut-brain connection, which is essential for a healthy digestive system, by stimulating the vagus nerve.

Practicing Meditation to Promote Gut Health

Reducing Stress: Meditation may help lessen the negative effects of stress on gut health by lowering cortisol levels. A greater knowledge of bodily signals, such as signs related to hunger and fullness, may also be fostered by practices such as mindfulness meditation.

Techniques for Mindfulness Meditation: Calming the mind and lessening gastrointestinal discomfort may be achieved with focused breathing techniques and guided visualization.

Effect on Microbiota: New study indicates that practicing meditation to decrease stress may benefit the makeup of the gut microbiota.

Including Meditation and Yoga in Everyday Life

Regular Practice: The secret is to develop a regular yoga and meditation schedule. For gut health, even brief daily activities may be quite beneficial.

Adaptability: Yoga is suitable for most people due to its ability to be tailored to different skill levels and physical conditions.

Resources & Guided Sessions: For novices, using internet resources or going to guided sessions may be beneficial in learning the right methods.

Evidence and Research from Science

Research on Yoga and Gut Health: A number of studies show that yoga may help with the symptoms of various digestive problems, such as irritable bowel syndrome (IBS).

Studies on Meditation: Studies on meditation have shown that it may be helpful for a number of illnesses that are made worse by stress, such as digestive ailments.

Obstacles and Safety Measures

Listening to the Body: It is important to avoid straining while doing yoga and meditation, particularly if you are experiencing severe gastrointestinal problems.

The Role of Sleep in Gut Health

Sleep is essential for preserving general health, which includes intestinal health.

Bidirectional Relationship: Sleep disorders may have a major effect on gut health, just as gut health can affect the quality of sleep. Inadequate sleep may affect the immune system, aggravate gastrointestinal diseases, and alter the gut microbiota.

Sleep and the Microbiome: Studies show that lack of sleep may change the makeup of gut flora, which may result in dysbiosis and related health problems.

Sleep Deprivation's Effects on Gut Health

Increased Inflammation: Sleep deprivation may lead to an increase in systemic inflammation, which can have a negative impact on gut health and perhaps exacerbate illnesses like irritable bowel syndrome (IBS) and inflammatory bowel disease (IBD).

Impaired Digestion and Absorption: Lack of sleep may interfere with the regular functioning of the digestive system, resulting in problems including acid reflux, indigestion, and hunger swings.

Stress and Gut Health: Insufficient sleep often results in high stress levels, which exacerbate digestive problems and symptoms.

Techniques to Enhance the Quality of Your Sleep

Consistent Sleep routine: Sleep quality is enhanced and the body's internal clock is regulated when a regular sleep routine is followed.

Establishing a sleep-inducing atmosphere in the bedroom which includes temperate temperatures, cozy bedding, and little light or noise can improve the quality of your sleep.

Reducing Stimulants: You may avoid sleep problems by avoiding coffee and large meals just before bed.

Relaxation Techniques: Before bed, engage in activities that help wind down and get the body ready for sleep, such as meditation, deep breathing, or mild yoga.

Sleep hygiene and alterations to one's lifestyle

Physical Activity: Exercise on a regular basis can enhance the quality of sleep, although it should be avoided just before bed.

Screen Time: Cutting down on blue light and screen time in the evening might aid in getting the body ready for sleep.

Mindful Eating: Eating a healthy, well-balanced diet that promotes gut health will also help you sleep better.

Effects of Particular Sleep Disorders on Digestive Health

Obstructive sleep apnea is one condition that may cause sleep disruption and negatively impact gut health.

Chronic insomnia may result in extended stress and worry, which can negatively affect gut health and general well-being.

6: Detoxification and Gut Health

Understanding Detoxification

The body naturally goes through a process called detoxification in order to neutralize, convert, and get rid of pollutants.

Definition and Objective: The term "detoxification" describes the natural cleaning and removal of waste materials and poisons by the body. It is a multisystemic, natural process that is ongoing and mostly affects the skin, lymphatic system, lungs, intestines, liver, and kidneys.

Toxicon Sources and Effects: In addition to internal sources like metabolic byproducts, toxins may also originate from external sources like chemicals, pollution, and bad diet.

The main detox organ is the liver.

Activities related to detoxification: The liver is essential for removing and filtering poisons. It changes harmful compounds into readily excreted nontoxic agents.

Liver detoxification phases: Liver detoxification occurs in two primary stages: Phase I, or transformation, and Phase II, or conjugation. Each stage uses a separate set of enzymes and physiological mechanisms.

The Gut's Function in Detoxification

Removal of Toxins: The removal of toxins is mostly dependent on the gut. Toxins and waste are effectively eliminated from the body when there is a healthy stomach and regular bowel movements.

Gut Microbiota and Detoxification: Toxins may be broken down and dangerous compounds can be protected against with the help of a healthy gut microbiome.

Skin, Lungs, and Kidneys in Detoxification

Kidneys: Remove toxins from the body via urine and filter blood.

Skin: Sweating gets rid of pollutants.

Lungs: Through breathing, release carbon dioxide and other volatile pollutants.

Nutrition and Elimination

Supportive Foods: A few foods, such as cruciferous vegetables, berries, garlic, and high-fiber diets, may help with the detoxification process.

Hydration: Drinking enough water is crucial for renal function and for making the removal of pollutants that dissolve in water easier.

Factors from Lifestyle That Affect Detoxification

Exercise: Increasing circulation and lymphatic drainage via regular physical exercise may help remove toxins.

Stress management: Prolonged stress may harm the digestive system and detoxification mechanisms.

Frequently Held Myths Regarding Detoxification

Detox Diets and Cleanses: Despite their widespread marketing, many detox diets and cleanses are unsupported by science and sometimes dangerous. For healthy people, the body's natural detoxification processes are usually enough.

Safe and Well-Being Detox Procedures

Modest Adjustments: Modest, lasting dietary and lifestyle adjustments are safer and more beneficial than drastic detoxification programs.

Consulting Healthcare Providers: This is crucial, especially for those who are ill or on medication.

Natural Detox Foods

The food plays a major role in assisting the body's natural detoxification processes. Some meals have a reputation for being detoxifying, improving liver function, nourishing the gastrointestinal tract, and facilitating the removal of toxins.

Foods that assist the body's natural detoxification processes fall under the category of natural detox foods. Antioxidants, fiber, vitamins, and minerals necessary for detoxification are usually found in these foods.

Their role in detoxification is multifaceted; they enhance the health of the gut flora, improve digestion, and support liver function.

Important Natural Detox Foods

Cruciferous Vegetables: Glucosinolates, found in broccoli, cauliflower, cabbage, and Brussels sprouts, aid in the liver's detoxification process.

Leafy Greens: Rich in chlorophyll, leafy greens like spinach, kale, and others may help cleanse the liver and digestive system.

Rich in sulfur-containing chemicals, garlic and onions aid in the liver's detoxification of a variety of toxins.

Berries: Rich in antioxidants, berries promote liver function by lowering oxidative stress.

Beets: Rich in minerals and antioxidants that support detoxification, beets are well-known for their ability to preserve the liver.

Green tea: Studies have shown that the antioxidants in it, called catechins, improve liver function.

Citrus Fruits: Vitamin C, which is abundant in lemons, limes, and oranges, aids in the transformation of poisons into water-soluble forms for simpler removal.

Apples: Packed with pectin, a fiber that helps clear the intestines and get rid of toxins.

Curcumin, an ingredient in turmeric, has anti-inflammatory and liver-protective qualities.

Ginger: Promotes liver health, aids with digestion, and relieves nausea.

Including Foods That Help You Reverse Diabetes

Balanced Meals: To aid in the body's natural detoxification processes, include a range of these detox foods in each meal.

Juices and smoothies are an easy approach to get a concentrated dose of nutrients that aid in detoxification.

Cooking Techniques: To retain the nutrients in these foods, steam, sauté, or roast them.

Frequent Intake: It's important to be consistent; including these items into your diet on a regular basis works better than drastic detoxification plans.

Dietary Guidelines and Safety Measures

Moderation and Variety: It's preferable to rely on a broad variety of detoxifying meals rather than ingesting too much of one kind.

Personal Intolerances: Take note of any allergies or dietary sensitivities.

Whenever feasible, go for organic options to reduce your exposure to chemicals and pesticides.

Safe Detox Practices

Detoxification is a popular idea, but it must be approached carefully and properly. The goal of detoxification should be to assist the body's natural detoxification processes rather than imposing severe food restrictions or using over-the-counter detox medications.

Definition: Safe detox techniques are dietary and lifestyle choices that, without harming the body or depleting it of nutrients, assist the body's natural cleansing organs such as the kidneys, liver, and gut.

Misconceptions: Detoxification is often misinterpreted as a fast cure or a speedy way to lose weight, which may result in unsafe and sometimes harmful behaviors.

Nutritional Methods for Safe Detoxification

Whole Foods: Make a diet high in unprocessed, whole foods your main focus. Fruits, vegetables, whole grains, lean meats, and good fats are all included in this.

Hydration: Getting enough water into your body is crucial for kidney health and aids in the removal of toxins that dissolve in water.

Fiber: Toxin and waste excretion depend on intestinal regularity, which is supported by a diet rich in fiber.

Reducing Toxin Intake: You may ease the strain on your detoxification systems by consuming less processed meals, alcoholic beverages, coffee, and sweets.

Lifestyle Changes to Help with Detoxification

Frequent Exercise: Exercise improves circulation and encourages sweating, which helps the skin expel pollutants.

Ensuring enough and high-quality sleep is essential for maintaining the body's natural detoxifying processes, particularly the regeneration cycle of the liver.

Stress management: You may lessen the negative effects of stress on your body's detoxifying organs by practicing yoga, meditation, and deep breathing.

Boosting Digestive Health for Clearing

Probiotics and Prebiotics: Effective detoxification depends on a healthy gut microbiota. Gut health may be supported by consuming foods high in probiotics and prebiotics.

Steer clear of unnecessary antibiotics: Gut flora may be disturbed by antibiotics. Use them under a doctor's supervision and only when medically required.

Utilizing Detox Supplements Safely

Consultation with Health Professionals: See a healthcare professional prior to beginning any supplement regimen, particularly if you are already taking medication or have pre-existing health concerns.

Natural Supplements: Take into account natural supplements with liver-supporting qualities, such as green tea, milk thistle, and dandelion.

Mental Health and Detox

Mind-Gut Connection: Recognize that physical health, including detoxification, depends on mental wellness.

Body positivity: Put more emphasis on wellbeing and health than on looks or weight reduction.

Observation and Modifications

Listen to Your Body: Be aware of how various detoxification techniques affect your body's response and make necessary adjustments.

Frequent medical examinations: Frequent check-ups with your doctor may help you track the impact of your detoxification regimen and avoid any negative health consequences.

Detox Myths Debunked

Myths and misunderstandings about detoxification are common in the field of health and wellbeing. To approach detoxification safely and efficiently, it's important to recognize the difference between prevalent beliefs and evidence-based treatments.

Myth 1: In order to detoxify, extreme diets are required.

The truth is that the liver, kidneys, and colon are the main detoxification organs that the human body has inbuilt mechanisms for. Not only are extreme detox diets needless, but they may also be dangerous, resulting in dietary deficits and other health issues.

Safe Method: The body's natural detoxification processes may be adequately supported by a balanced diet high in fruits, vegetables, whole grains, and lean proteins.

Myth 2: Pricey Supplements and Detox Products Are Necessary

Reality: A lot of over-the-counter detox and supplement products provide more marketing than real health advantages. The effectiveness of these products in helping the body detoxify is not well supported by scientific research.

Safe Approach: Put your attention on detoxifying naturally with food, water, exercise, and rest. Be sure to speak with a doctor before taking any supplements.

Myth 3: Losing Weight Quickly with Detoxification

Reality: Detox diets are not long-term, healthy weight reduction plans, even if they might provide temporary weight loss owing to water loss or calorie restriction in some cases.

Safe Approach: For healthy and long-term weight control, adopt a balanced diet and frequent exercise.

Myth 4: Certain Foods and Beverages Help the Body "Detox"

Reality: The body cannot "detox" from a single meal or beverage. The process of detoxification is intricately regulated by the body's organs and is not linked to any particular diet or drink.

Safe Method: Consume a wide range of meals high in nutrients to support your body's natural detoxification processes as well as your general wellness.

Myth 5: The Gut Can Remove Toxins with a Detox Diet

Truth: Regular bowel movements allow the intestines to naturally remove waste and poisons. Severe detoxification regimens have the potential to damage rather than help the native gut flora.

Safe Approach: Eat foods high in probiotics, drink plenty of water, and follow a high-fiber diet to keep your gut healthy.

Myth 6: Regular Detoxing Is Health Benefiting

Reality: Consistently putting the body through harsh detoxification regimens or fasting may cause nutritional deficits, muscular atrophy, and metabolic disturbances, among other health problems.

Safe Approach: Prioritize regular healthy diet and lifestyle choices over sporadic detoxifications.

Myth 7: Lifestyle Choices Unhealthy Can Be Made Whole Again Through Detoxification

The truth is that detoxification cannot replace leading a healthy lifestyle. Periodic detoxification cannot offset regular use of tobacco products, alcohol, or poor eating habits.

Safe Approach: Take a comprehensive approach to well-being, including regular exercise, a nutritious diet, and abstaining from drugs.

7: Gut Health through the Lifespan

Gut Health in Adolescence

Significant changes occur throughout the teenage years on the physical, psychological, and emotional levels, all of which are impacted by and affected by the gut.

Physiological Changes: Hormonal changes brought on by puberty throughout adolescence may have an impact on gut function. It is also around this time when the gut microbiota matures.

Dietary Habits: Teens often have more control over what they eat, which may result in eating habits that are either healthy or unhealthy and negatively impact gut health.

Adolescents' Gut Health Obstacles

Increased Risk of Disorders: Adolescence is generally the time when conditions like eating disorders and irritable bowel syndrome (IBS), which may impact gut health, initially manifest or worsen.

Stress and Anxiety: Through the gut-brain axis, stresses that are typical of adolescence, such as social dynamics and academic expectations, may affect gut health.

Dietary Elements That Affect Gut Health

Balanced Diet: A gut microbiota that is in good health is supported by a diet high in fruits, vegetables, whole grains, and lean meats.

Fast food and processed foods: Eating a lot of these items may have a bad effect on gut health and cause problems including bloating, diarrhea, and constipation.

Hydration: Drinking enough water is crucial to maintaining a healthy digestive system and avoiding constipation.

The Significance of Exercise

Exercise and Gut Motility: Engaging in regular physical exercise helps enhance gut health and motility.

Exercise is a powerful stress reliever that also has a knock-on effect on intestinal health.

Gut and Mental Health

Emotional Well-Being: Since stress, worry, and depression may have a major negative influence on gut health, it is important to address mental health.

Coping mechanisms include practicing mindfulness, meditation, and taking up activities that promote gut health and stress management.

Aspects of Education

Understanding Gut Health: Teaching teenagers the value of gut health and how it affects general wellbeing might promote better lifestyle choices.

Programs centered in schools: Adolescents' gut health may be supported by implementing instructional programs in schools that emphasize physical exercise, nutrition, and mental health.

Early Intervention and Preventive Action

Frequent check-ups: Tracking growth and development throughout adolescence may aid in the early detection and treatment of any disorders related to gut health.

Support from Parents and Caregivers: It's critical that parents and caregivers take an active role in encouraging good diet and lifestyle choices.

Pregnancy and Gut Health

Significant physiological changes occur during pregnancy, many of which have an effect on gut health.

Changes in Gut Health during Pregnancy

Hormonal Influences: Progesterone in particular during pregnancy has the ability to relax the muscles in the digestive system, which may cause delayed digestion and frequent problems like acid reflux and constipation.

Physical Changes: As the fetus develops, pain in the gastrointestinal tract may be caused in part by increasing abdominal pressure.

Typical Digestive Problems during Pregnancy

Morning Sickness: During the first trimester in particular, nausea and vomiting are frequent and may have an impact on the health of the stomach and the absorption of nutrients.

Constipation: During pregnancy, a reduction in intestinal motility often causes constipation.

Acid reflux and heartburn may be caused by changes in hormones and increased abdominal pressure, which is known as gastroesophageal reflux disease (GERD).

The Gut Microbiota's Function during Pregnancy

Maternal Microbiome: Modifications to the gut microbiome during gestation may have an effect on the health of the mother and the course of the pregnancy.

Impact on Fetal Development: According to recently conducted study, the mother's gut microbiota may have an impact on the health of her unborn child as well as fetal development.

Dietary Guidelines for Pregnancy-Related Gut Health

Fiber-Rich Diet: Eating a diet rich in whole grains, legumes, fruits, and vegetables might help ease constipation.

Hydration: Drinking more water is crucial to promoting healthy digestion and avoiding constipation.

Smaller, More Often Meals: Eating more often spaced out meals will help control nausea and lessen the likelihood of acid reflux.

Probiotics and Supplements

Prenatal vitamins are crucial for addressing dietary requirements that may not be satisfied by food alone.

Probiotics: Selecting strains that are safe during pregnancy might be crucial in maintaining a healthy gut flora.

Exercise and Gut Health

Safe Exercise: Taking part in safe workouts during pregnancy might help with constipation and digestion.

Pelvic Floor Health: Building strength in the pelvic floor may assist prepare the body for delivery and help manage some gastrointestinal problems.

Controlling Stress and Maintaining Gut Health

Mind-Body Techniques: Stress management is a benefit for both the mental and digestive health of expectant mothers. Techniques like prenatal yoga and meditation may aid with this.

Medical Advice and Supervision

Frequent Checkups: It's essential to have ongoing medical treatment to check the health of both the mother and the fetus.

Handling GI Disorders: You should speak with a healthcare professional about any severe or enduring gastrointestinal problems.

Menopause and Microbiome Changes

Menstrual cycles ending and major hormonal changes, especially a decrease in estrogen levels, are hallmarks of menopause, a normal stage in a woman's life. The gut microbiota is one of the many elements of health that may be significantly impacted by these modifications.

Hormonal Fluctuations: The immune system, gut motility, and barrier function are all impacted by the decline in estrogen that occurs during menopause, and these factors all contribute to gut health.

Hormonal changes during menopause may affect the makeup of the gut microbiota. This can have an influence on general health and increase the risk of postmenopausal illnesses such as cardiovascular disease and osteoporosis.

Common Menopausal Gut-Related Problems

Enhanced Vulnerability to GI Disorders: Menopause may cause changes in the symptomatology or development of conditions such as irritable bowel syndrome (IBS) and inflammatory bowel disease (IBD).

Bloating and Constipation: Problems like bloating and constipation may be brought on by abnormalities in gastrointestinal motility.

Weight Gain and Metabolic Changes: Hormone fluctuations may impact body composition and metabolism, which in turn can impact gut health.

Dietary Techniques for Menopausal Gut Health

Consumption of Fiber: In order to keep the digestive tract motile and avoid constipation, a diet rich in fiber is essential.

Plant-based foods that contain phytoestrogens, such as soy products, may help to balance hormones.

Vitamin D and calcium are essential for healthy bones, particularly after menopause. Since the gut is where these nutrients are absorbed, good gut health is necessary for optimal nutrient utilization.

Foods High in Probiotics and Prebiotics: A healthy gut environment may be maintained by providing prebiotic fibers and fermented foods to support the gut bacteria.

Changes in Lifestyle

Frequent Exercise: Exercise helps control weight, enhance gastrointestinal motility, and lower the incidence of menopausal-related chronic illnesses.

Hydration: Keeping the gut healthy overall and avoiding constipation depend on consuming enough fluids.

Stress management: Menopause-related stress may have an adverse effect on gut health. Methods like yoga, meditation, and mindfulness can assist.

Gut Health with Hormone Replacement Therapy (HRT)

Gut Microbiome Impact: Although its effects are diverse and unique to each person, hormone replacement therapy (HRT) may affect the composition and function of the gut microbiota.

Considering and Consulting: Given that HRT may have an effect on gut health, it is crucial to discuss the advantages and disadvantages of the treatment with a healthcare professional.

Observation and Medical Assistance

Frequent Health Check-ups: Monitoring digestive health and general well-being with routine check-ups both before and after menopause.

Expert Dietary Advice: Getting individualized dietary advice from a nutritionist to address digestive problems associated with menopause.

Aging and Gut Health

Our bodies change with age in many ways, and the stomach is no exception. The gut microbiota and digestive system are highly impacted by aging, which may have an impact on general health and quality of life.

The Effects of Aging on Gut Health

Physiological Changes: The digestive system normally slows down as we age, which affects the motility and functionality of the stomach. The immune system, bowel habits, and nutrition absorption may all be impacted by these modifications.

Alterations in the Gut Microbiome: As people age, their gut microbiota's diversity and composition tend to shift, which may have an effect on anything from immunological response to digestion.

Typical Digestive Problems in Seniors

One of the most prevalent GI problems in the elderly is constipation, which is often brought on by decreased gut motility, a decline in physical activity, and adverse drug reactions.

Diverticular Disease: Diverticular disease is caused by the colon wall deteriorating with age.

Reduced esophageal motility and hiatal hernia are two variables that contribute to the increased incidence of gastroesophageal reflux disease (GERD) in older persons.

Malabsorption: As people age, their body's capacity to absorb certain nutrients, such calcium, iron, and vitamin B12, may decline.

Dietary Factors Associated with Aging Gut Health

High-Fiber Diet: To avoid constipation and preserve a healthy gut microbiota, a diet high in fiber from fruits, vegetables, and whole grains is essential.

Sufficient Fluid Intake: Digestion and constipation prevention depend on consuming enough fluids.

Nutrient-Dense Foods: To help with malabsorption and promote general health, emphasize foods rich in vitamins, minerals, and antioxidants.

Mindful Eating: Observing signs of hunger and fullness, as aging may alter how the body regulates appetite.

Lifestyle Factors Affecting Aging Gut Health

Frequent Exercise: Keeping an active lifestyle helps enhance digestive health in general and intestinal motility in particular.

Stress management: Stress management is good for gut health and may be achieved by practices like yoga, meditation, or taking up a hobby.

Senior Diets: Prebiotics and Probiotics

Probiotics' role: Eating foods high in probiotics, such as kefir, yogurt, and fermented vegetables, may help maintain a balanced gut flora.

Prebiotic Foods: Foods high in prebiotics, such as onions, garlic, and bananas, support healthy gut flora.

Taking Care of Drug Side Effects

Examining medicines: It's important to routinely check medicines with a healthcare professional since some, especially those that alter bowel movements or acid production, may have a detrimental effect on gut health.

Health Monitoring and Proactive Treatment

Frequent Check-Ups: Regular check-ups may aid in monitoring gut health and identifying any problems early on.

Making a GI Disorder Screening: following guidelines for suggested tests to identify and prevent gastrointestinal disorders, such as colonoscopies.

Choosing the Right Probiotics

By keeping the gut microbiome in balance, probiotics also known as "good" or "friendly" bacteria play a critical role in preserving gut health. Selecting the best probiotic pill or meal might be overwhelming due to the wide range of options available.

Definition: Probiotics are living microorganisms that provide the host health benefits when given in sufficient doses.

Probiotic Strain Types: Lactobacillus, Bifidobacterium, and Saccharomyces are common probiotic microorganisms that each have unique functions and advantages for gut health.

Probiotic Advantages

Gut Health: By maintaining the proper balance of gut microbiota, they support immunological, digestive, and nutritional absorption processes.

Probiotics have been shown to be useful in both avoiding and lessening the severity of diarrhea brought on by illnesses or the use of antibiotics.

Handling Irritable Bowel Syndrome (IBS): Certain strains have the ability to reduce IBS symptoms.

Support for the Immune System: They may strengthen defenses against infections and boost immunity.

Considerations for Selecting Probiotics

Certain Strains for Certain Needs: The advantages of various strains vary. It's critical to choose a probiotic that meets specific health demands, such as immune system support, allergy control, or gut health.

Choose probiotic strains that have undergone clinical studies and have efficacious proof to back them up.

Units for Forming Colonies (CFUs): The number of CFUs in a probiotic is often used to determine its efficacy. The effective dosage varies depending on the strain in question and the ailment being treated, thus more CFUs are not necessarily better.

Quality and Purity: Select probiotics from reliable companies that follow high standards in their production processes.

Probiotic Supplements vs. Foods

Probiotic Foods: As part of a balanced diet, fermented foods such as kimchi, kefir, sauerkraut, and yogurt naturally contain probiotics.

Supplements: There are many different kinds of probiotic supplements, including as capsules, pills, and powders. They may provide concentrated concentrations of certain strains that are not usually found in dietary sources.

Guidelines for Probiotic Supplementation

Consulting Medical Experts: See a doctor before taking any probiotic supplements, particularly if you have any underlying medical issues or are already taking other drugs.

Keeping and Managing: Observe the storage guidelines, since some probiotic supplements may need to be refrigerated in order to stay effective.

Course Length: While some probiotics are taken for a set amount of time, others may be included in the diet on a daily basis.

Prebiotic Supplements

Prebiotics are just as vital but often less understood than probiotics, despite probiotics receiving a lot of attention for their health advantages. Dietary fibers known as prebiotics nourish the good bacteria in the stomach.

Recognizing Prebiotics

Prebiotics are defined as non-digestible dietary ingredients, mainly fibers and oligosaccharides that stimulate the development and function of good gut flora.

Their function is to feed probiotics, which in turn helps to maintain a balanced and healthy gut microbiota.

Different Prebiotic Supplement Types

Inulin: A common prebiotic fiber present in a wide variety of plants, inulin is used in supplements often because it effectively promotes the development of gut bacteria that are good to the body.

Short fructose chains known as fructo-oligosaccharides (FOS) serve as prebiotic fibers.

Galacto-oligosaccharides (GOS): These lactose-derived molecules are known to specifically support Bifidobacteria in the gastrointestinal tract.

Foods such as unripe bananas and boiled and cooled potatoes contain resistant starch, which functions as a prebiotic and withstands digestion.

Advantages of Supplemental Prebiotics

Gut Health: Prebiotics help maintain a balanced microbiota in the gut, which is essential for immunological response, nutrition absorption, and digestion.

Digestive Comfort: They may support regular bowel motions and help fend against constipation.

Metabolic Health: Prebiotics may help with weight control, blood sugar regulation, and satiety by influencing these parameters, according to some research.

The Appropriate Prebiotic Supplement Selection

Source and Quality: Seek for premium supplements that list the kind and quantity of prebiotic fiber they include.

Probiotic Complementation: To achieve a synergistic impact, take prebiotics together with probiotics.

Consulting Medical Experts: particularly crucial for those on restricted diets or those suffering from digestive issues.

How to Include Prebiotics in Your Diet

Gradual Introduction: To prevent bloating or discomfort as the gut flora responds to higher fiber, start with a modest dosage and increase it gradually.

Food Sources: For a more organic intake, combine supplements with food sources of prebiotics such garlic, onions, leeks, asparagus, and bananas.

Consistency: Keeping the gut healthy requires consistently consuming prebiotics.

Things to Think About and Potential Side Effects

Individual Tolerance: When introducing prebiotics for the first time, some persons may suffer pain, bloating, or gas. This is often transient and may be reduced with a slow introduction.

Drug Interactions: There may be drug interactions between certain prebiotic supplements and specific drugs. It's crucial to talk about this with a medical professional.

Vitamins and Minerals for Gut Health

Although the importance of vitamins and minerals in preserving general health is well recognized, their precise influence on intestinal health cannot be overstated.

Essential Vitamins for Digestive Health

Vitamin D: Is essential for both immunological response and gut lining health. Reduced vitamin D levels have been linked to a higher risk of intestinal inflammation and conditions such as inflammatory bowel disease (IBD).

Vitamin A: Essential for immune system performance and preserving the integrity of the gut lining. Foods high in it include sweet potatoes, carrots, and leafy greens.

Vitamin B: B vitamins are necessary for cellular activity and the healing of the intestinal lining, particularly B12 and folate. Meat, dairy products, eggs, and fortified cereals all contain them.

Vital Minerals for Digestive Health

Zinc: Required for immunological system and gut lining repair. A zinc shortage may result in a "leaky gut" an increase in intestinal permeability. Meat, seafood, legumes, and seeds are examples of sources.

Magnesium: Found in foods including leafy greens, nuts, seeds, and whole grains, magnesium is involved in several digestive processes and may help control bowel motions.

Iron: Essential for the body's oxygen delivery system. Iron deficiency is often seen in diseases such as celiac disease and may have an influence on gut health. Fish, chicken, red meat, and fortified grains are examples of rich sources.

Mineral and vitamin supplements

When to Supplement: When food intake is inadequate or when there are circumstances where there are greater needs such as with certain medical conditions or aging supplements may be required.

Selecting Supplements: Selecting premium supplements and seeking advice from a healthcare provider are crucial, especially to prevent overindulgence that may be hazardous.

Minerals and Vitamins' Function in the Microbiome

Microbial Development: The development of good gut bacteria may be influenced by certain vitamins and minerals, which can have an effect on gut health in general.

Digestive Enzymes: The synthesis of digestive enzymes requires sufficient amounts of a few specific vitamins and minerals.

Interactions between Drugs

Possible Interactions: The efficacy of certain drugs may be altered by interactions with certain vitamins and minerals. It's crucial to talk to your healthcare physician about supplement usage.

Lifestyle and Nutritional Factors

Balanced Diet: Most people can acquire all the vitamins and minerals they need for gut health by eating a diet high in whole grains, fruits, vegetables, lean meats, and healthy fats.

Cooking Techniques That Are Gut-Friendly: Roasting or boiling food helps retain its nutritional value.

Herbal Remedies for Digestive Health

For millennia, people have utilized herbal treatments to address a variety of digestive problems. Knowing how certain herbs might support digestive wellbeing is more important than ever, as interest in alternative health treatments grows.

Essential Herbs for a Healthy Stomach

Ginger: Known for its ability to reduce nausea, ginger also relieves bloating, gas, and stomach symptoms. It helps with moderate stomach distress and promotes digestion.

Peppermint: Well-known for its antispasmodic qualities, peppermint helps ease IBS symptoms, calm the digestive system, and lessen pain in the abdomen.

Chamomile: Known for its anti-inflammatory and relaxing properties, chamomile may ease minor digestive pain, lessen the impact of stress on digestive problems, and encourage relaxation.

Dandelion: The leaves and roots help the liver and digestive system. Additionally, dandelion may support a balanced gut microbiota.

Licorice Root: Known to calm the stomach lining and lessen inflammation, licorice root is often used in situations of gastritis and heartburn. It is advised to use deglycyrrhizinated licorice (DGL) in order to prevent any possible glycyrrhizin adverse effects.

Slippery elm: It helps with GERD, gastritis, and ulcers by creating a calming film across the lining of the digestive system.

Fennel: Often used to treat indigestion, fennel is well-known for its carminative qualities. It may also alleviate gas and bloating.

Turmeric: This root vegetable contains curcumin, an antioxidant and anti-inflammatory compound that is good for the stomach and reduces inflammation in general.

Including Herbal Remedies in Your Nutrition

Teas and Infusions: Herbs used in digestion may be drunk as teas. Peppermint tea, for instance, may help with digestion after meals.

Cooking: Adding herbs like turmeric and ginger to food improves taste and is good for the digestive system.

Supplements: More concentrated dosages of herbal supplements are available, but they should only be used under a doctor's supervision.

Safety and Things to Think About

Drug Interactions: A number of botanicals have the potential to interact with prescription drugs. It's important to speak with a doctor before beginning any herbal treatment.

Purity and Quality: Select premium organic herbal items to guarantee effectiveness and purity.

Allergies and Side Effects: Take precautions against possible allergies and begin with low dosages to watch for any negative responses.

Personal Requirements and Preferences

Personalized Approach: Everybody responds differently to various herbs. To determine what is most effective for you, you may need to experiment a little.

Integration with Other Therapies: When combined with dietary and lifestyle modifications, herbal medicines may provide a holistic strategy for digestive health.

9: Gut Health and Weight Management

Gut Microbiome and Obesity

The gut microbiota and obesity are significantly correlated, according to recent study, which has changed our knowledge of how to control weight.

Definition and Make-Up: The billions of bacteria, viruses, and fungi that live in the gastrointestinal system are collectively referred to as the gut microbiome. Every person has a different makeup, which is determined by a variety of variables including genetics, lifestyle, and nutrition.

Function in Health: These microbes are essential for proper digestion, nutritional absorption, immunological response, and even mood and behavior modulation.

The Relationship between Obesity and Gut Microbiota

Microbiota Diversity: Studies show that compared to people of normal weight, obese people often have a less varied gut microbiome.

Effect on Metabolism: The rate at which energy is derived from meals and the amount of fat that is stored in the body may both be affected by certain gut flora.

Obesity and Inflammation: Metabolic diseases and obesity are linked to low-grade chronic inflammation, which may be caused by dysbiosis, or an imbalance in the gut microbiota.

Mechanisms Connecting Obesity and Gut Microbiota

Short-Chain Fatty Acids (SCFAs): Regulating hunger and energy metabolism are two of the effects of SCFAs, which are produced when gut bacteria digest food fibers.

Leaky Gut Syndrome: Elevated intestinal permeability may cause systemic inflammation, which in turn can exacerbate insulin resistance and weight gain.

Gut Hormones: Hormones that control hunger and fullness, such as ghrelin and leptin, are secreted in response to interactions with gut flora.

Food Repercussions on the Gut Microbiota

Diets heavy in fat and low in fiber: These may encourage the development of microorganisms linked to obesity.

Probiotics and Prebiotics: Eating foods high in these microorganisms helps support the maintenance of a balanced gut microbiota, which may have an impact on how well people control their weight.

Balanced, diversified Diet: Eating a diet high in fruits, vegetables, whole grains, and lean meats can help to support a healthy, diversified gut microbiota.

Environmental and Lifestyle Factors

Physical Activity: The variety and makeup of the gut microbiome may be favorably impacted by regular exercise.

Antibiotics and Medications: Some drugs have the potential to alter the gut flora, which may affect metabolism and weight.

Interventions and Therapy

Personalized nutrition: Adapting dietary treatments to a person's gut microbiota may be a more successful strategy for controlling obesity.

Probiotic and prebiotic supplements: Although studies are still being conducted, these supplements may be able to influence the gut flora in order to treat obesity.

Dieting and Gut Health

Dieting has a complicated and multidimensional relationship with gut health, especially when it comes to weight reduction. Comprehending the effects of diverse meals on the gut flora and general digestive health is crucial for efficient and long-lasting weight control.

Dietary Effects on the Gut Microbiota

Dietary Changes: A substantial shift in diet has the potential to alter the gut microbiome's makeup. For example, diets heavy in fat and low in carbohydrates may decrease the variety of bacteria.

Calorie Restriction: Although cutting calories might help you lose weight, it can also affect how many good bacteria are in your stomach.

Gut Health-Promoting Dietary Practices

A balanced diet that prioritizes consuming the right amounts of micronutrients and macronutrients (fats, proteins, and carbs) to promote gut health and weight control.

High-Fiber Foods: A diet high in fruits, vegetables, legumes, and whole grains may help control weight and support a healthy gut microbiota.

Probiotics and Prebiotics: Eating foods high in prebiotics (garlic, onions, and bananas) and probiotics (yogurt and kefir) may help maintain a healthy gut environment while losing weight.

Steer Clear of Fad Diets for Gut Health

Short-Term Gains, Long-Term Losses: While fad diets may provide rapid weight reduction, they may also cause nutritional shortages and disruptions in the gut microbiota.

Sustainability: It is better to concentrate on long-term, sustainable dietary habits for gut health and weight control.

Digestive Health and Mindful Eating

Awareness and Regulation: Eating mindfully improves digestion and fosters a positive connection with food by raising awareness of hunger and fullness signals.

Stress reduction: Lowering the amount of stress associated with eating decisions may improve general wellbeing and gut health.

Dietary Practices' Effects on Gut Health

Ketogenic Diet: Although it may help with weight reduction, it can also alter the makeup of gut flora. Vegetables high in fiber and low in carbohydrates may help lessen this.

Plant-Based Diets: Because they include a lot of fiber, these diets are generally good for gut health, but it's vital to make sure you're getting enough protein.

Intermittent fasting: May improve metabolic health and have a positive impact on the makeup of the gut microbiota.

Hydration's Significance for Gut Health and Dieting

Sufficient Water Consumption: Crucial for healthy digestion and gut regularity, particularly when consuming more fiber.

Supplementing While on a Diet

Multivitamins and Minerals: To avoid deficiency while on a diet low in calories.

Probiotic supplements: May be useful to maintain gut health, especially if dietary probiotic use is restricted.

Exercise and Metabolic Health

The key to preserving metabolic health, which is essential for managing weight, is exercise. Physical exercise has a major influence on gut health and metabolic processes in addition to its well-known advantages for cardiovascular health and muscular strength.

Exercise's Significance for Metabolic Health

Improving Metabolic Rate: Engaging in regular physical exercise raises metabolic rate, which aids in calorie burning even while at rest.

Enhancing Insulin Sensitivity: Physical activity lowers the risk of metabolic diseases including type 2 diabetes by increasing the body's sensitivity to insulin.

Hormone Regulation: Exercise has a role in controlling appetite and satiety-promoting hormones like leptin and ghrelin.

The Effects of Exercise on Gut Health

Variety of Gut Microbiota: Research has shown that consistent exercise enhances gut microbiota diversity, which is associated with better health outcomes.

Improved Gut Motility: Physical activity may help the digestive system operate better, which helps lessen bloating and constipation symptoms.

Stress Reduction: Exercise may help create a better gut environment by lowering stress, which is known to have a detrimental impact on gut health.

Exercise Types for Metabolic Health

Aerobic Exercise: Exercises that improve cardiovascular health and burn calories include cycling, swimming, walking, and running.

Strength Training: Strength training increases muscular mass, which improves body composition and increases metabolic rate.

High-Intensity Interval Training (HIIT): Improving metabolic health may be very successfully accomplished by short bursts of high exercise interspersed with rest intervals.

Including Exercise in Plans for Weight Management

Consistency: Gaining metabolic advantages from exercise requires regular, consistent activity.

Customized Exercise Programs: Creating an exercise schedule based on a person's objectives, preferences, and degree of fitness.

Blending Nutrition with Exercise: The most successful weight control strategies include regular physical exercise with a nutritious diet.

Overcoming Obstacles to Physical Activity

Time Restrictions: You may get around time constraints by finding methods to include physical exercise into your everyday routine, like riding your bike or walking to work.

Motivation: Getting regular exercisers motivated may be enhanced by setting attainable objectives, monitoring their progress, and looking for social support.

Physical Restrictions: Modifying workouts to account for any physical restrictions or medical issues, and seeking medical advice as required.

10: Building a Gut-Healthy Lifestyle

Creating a Balanced Diet Plan

Maintaining gut health, which in turn affects general health and well-being, requires a balanced diet.

The Essentials of a Diet for Gut Health

Variety of Foods: Eating a variety diet full of whole grains, lean meats, fruits, veggies, and healthy fats guarantees a broad range of nutrients and supports a diverse gut microbiota.

High Intake of Fiber: Fiber feeds the good bacteria in the gut and is necessary for regular bowel movements. Whole grains, legumes, fruits, and vegetables are examples of sources.

Probiotic Foods: Foods that provide good bacteria to the stomach include kefir, yogurt, sauerkraut, and kimchi.

Prebiotic foods: These include foods like garlic, onions, bananas, and asparagus that nourish good gut flora.

Making a Diet Plan That Is Balanced

Personalization: Adapting the diet plan to each person's tastes, way of life, and nutritional requirements while taking their age, degree of activity, and health objectives into account.

Control Your Portion Size: Eating the right amounts of food will help you stay at a healthy weight and avoid gastrointestinal distress.

Hydration: Drinking enough water is essential for proper digestion and absorption of nutrients.

Addition of Nutrient-Dense Foods

Whole Foods: For the highest nutritional content, emphasize whole, unprocessed foods.

Lean Proteins: For the upkeep and regeneration of muscles, include foods like fish, chicken, beans, and tofu.

Healthy Fats: Because of their anti-inflammatory qualities, fats may be obtained from foods including avocados, nuts, seeds, and olive oil.

Macronutrient Equilibrium

Carbohydrates: For long-lasting energy and intestinal health, choose complex carbs like whole grains.

Proteins: Making sure you eat enough protein to support immunological and tissue repair processes.

Fats: Because they aid in nutrition absorption and satiety, include healthy fats in your diet.

Steer Clear of Gut Irritants

Cut Back on Processed Foods: Processed meals, which are poor in nutrients and high in additives, may harm the stomach.

Cutting Back on Sugar and Alcohol: Overindulgence in these substances may cause disruptions in the microbiota of the stomach.

Be Aware of Sensitivities to Food: being conscious of one's own dietary intolerances or sensitivities, such as lactose or gluten, and modifying one's diet appropriately.

Planning and Preparing Meals

Regular Meal Times: Eating at regular intervals might help the digestive system operate regularly.

Cooking at home allows you to have more control over the ingredients and cooking techniques.

Trying new dishes: To keep the diet interesting and varied, try different dishes.

Integrating Physical Activity

Exercise is great for cardiovascular health and general fitness, but it's also very important for gut health maintenance.

The Connection between Gut Health and Physical Activity

Increased Diversity of the Gut Microbiome: It has been shown that regular exercise increases the diversity of the gut microbiome, which is essential for gut health and general wellbeing.

Better Digestion and Gut Motility: By encouraging the natural contraction of the digestive muscles, physical exercise helps enhance digestion and guard against problems like constipation.

Stress Reduction: Physical exercise indirectly helps the digestive tract since stress may have a detrimental effect on gut health. Exercise is also a very effective stress reliever.

Exercise Types That Are Good for Gut Health

Aerobic exercises: Exercises like jogging, cycling, swimming, and walking help improve gut motility and enhance blood flow to the digestive system.

Strength Training: Increasing muscular mass enhances metabolism generally, which may benefit intestinal health.

Pilates and yoga are two types of exercise that not only help people decompress but also have certain positions and motions that may improve digestion and ease pain.

Including Exercise in Everyday Activities

Frequent Exercise Regimen: Creating a regular exercise schedule based on personal preferences and fitness levels.

Including Physical Activity in Everyday Life: Making little adjustments like using the stairs, biking or walking to work, or taking up active hobbies may all add up to more total physical activity.

Fun Activities: To guarantee long-term commitment, choose fun fitness programs.

Getting Past Obstacles to Exercise

Time management is the art of scheduling and prioritizing physical activity to make time for exercise in a hectic schedule.

Commencing Small: For those who are not used to exercising often, begin with easy-to-manage exercises and progressively increase the time and intensity.

Looking for Expert Advice: seeking advice from physical therapists or fitness experts, particularly for those with certain health issues or physical restrictions.

Exercise and Nutritional Factors

Keeping the right amount of water in your body, especially before, during, and after exercise.

Nutrient Timing: Fueling the body and promoting recovery before and after exercise with well-balanced meals and snacks.

Assessing Exercise's Effect on Gut Health

Keeping an eye on digestive changes observing changes in gut health or digestion while establishing or modifying workout regimens.

Adapting as required: being willing to modify exercise regimens and levels of intensity in response to gut health and comfort levels.

Stress Reduction Techniques
Stress may significantly affect gut health and be a factor in a variety of gastrointestinal problems. Thus, cultivating a gut-healthy lifestyle requires effective stress management.

Knowing How Stress Affects the Gut

Stress has an impact on the gut-brain axis, a sophisticated communication system that regulates gut motility, secretion, and microbial balance between the brain and digestive tract.

Effect on Digestive Health: Prolonged stress may result in gastrointestinal tract inflammation, ulcers, and IBS, among other digestive issues.

Practical Methods for Reducing Stress

Stress and its effects on the stomach may be lessened by practicing mindfulness meditation, which is concentrating on the here and now while accepting thoughts and emotions without passing judgment.

Deep Breathing Exercises: By triggering the body's relaxation response, techniques such as diaphragmatic breathing may reduce stress and perhaps even enhance intestinal health.

Yoga and Tai Chi are mind-body exercises that incorporate breathing exercises, physical postures, and meditation to lower stress and improve intestinal health.

Progressive muscle relaxation, or PMR, is a technique that helps release physical tension and stress by first tensing and then releasing various muscle groups.

Frequent Exercise

Exercise as a Stress Reliever: Regular physical exercise, such as cycling, swimming, or walking, may dramatically lower stress levels and enhance gut health inadvertently.

Nature Exposure: Engaging in outdoor activities that require spending time in nature, such as gardening or hiking, might further improve stress reduction.

Sustaining Social Relationships

Support Systems: Social interactions and solid connections may provide emotional support, which can aid in stress management.

Community Involvement: Volunteering or taking part in activities held in the community may give one a sense of direction and lessen stress.

Optimal Sleep Practices

The significance of sleep: Getting enough rest is essential for stress management. It is crucial to practice proper sleep hygiene, which includes keeping a regular sleep schedule and setting up a relaxing atmosphere.

Methods of Relaxation: The quality of your sleep may be enhanced by including relaxing activities before bed, such as reading or having a warm bath.

Stress and Diet

A balanced diet that is high in whole foods and includes plenty of fruits, vegetables, and whole grains may provide you the nutrients you need to manage stress.

Reducing sugar and caffeine consumption, which may worsen stress and have an impact on gut health, is known as "limiting stimulants."

Long-Term Gut Health Strategies
Sustaining gut health is a lifelong journey, not a short-term goal.

Basis of a Diet for Gut Health

Regular Good Eating Practices: A well-balanced diet high in fiber, lean meats, healthy fats, probiotics, and prebiotics ought to be a regular part of a person's daily diet.

Diversity in Food Choices: Eating a diverse range of meals on a regular basis guarantees a broad spectrum of nutrients and fosters a diverse gut microbiota.

Moderation and Mindfulness: To prevent overindulging and upset stomach, practice moderation in portion sizes and mindfulness while selecting foods.

Frequent Exercise

Exercise Consistency: Sticking to a regular exercise schedule that suits individual needs and abilities.

Including Physical Activity in Lifestyle: Identifying methods to maintain an active lifestyle, such as climbing the stairs, walking or cycling to work, or participating in leisure activities or hobbies.

Stress Reduction

Regular stress-reduction techniques include deep breathing exercises, yoga, meditation, and stress-relieving hobbies.

Work-Life Harmony: actively controlling one's personal and professional life to minimize chronic stress, which has a negative impact on gut health.

Sleep and Hydration

Adequate Water Intake: Maintaining a steady and adequate level of hydration to aid in digestion and general well-being.

Good sleep hygiene should be followed, and sleep problems should be quickly resolved since insufficient sleep may negatively affect gut health.

Frequent Medical Exams

Regular medical monitoring include regular check-ups with medical specialists that include testing and screenings related to digestive health.

A proactive approach to digestive issues involves seeing a doctor about any persistent or worrisome symptoms related to the digestive system.

Continual Education and Adjustment

Keeping Up: Keeping abreast of the most recent findings and suggestions about gut health.

Adapting to Life Changes: During various life phases, such as pregnancy, menopause, or aging, gut health methods should be modified as required.

Creating a Community of Support

Social Connections: Keeping up solid social relationships has been linked to improved intestinal and mental health.

Engaging with communities or organizations that are focused on gut health and healthy living is one way to share knowledge and experiences.

Utilizing Supplements and Medications Mindfully

Antibiotic Use: Use with Caution: Since antibiotics might alter gut flora, only use them when absolutely required.

Supplements as Needed: Taking into account supplements, such fiber or probiotics, in accordance with personal requirements and expert advice.

11: Overcoming Challenges in Gut Health

Dealing with Food Sensitivities

The gut lining and general health may be greatly impacted by food sensitivities and intolerances. Maintaining a healthy digestive system requires knowing how to recognize and handle these sensitivities.

Knowing Your Food Sensitivities

Types and Definition: Unlike food allergies, food sensitivities or intolerances are unpleasant responses to certain foods that do not involve the immune system. Typical instances include gluten sensitivity and lactose intolerance.

Signs: might include less severe symptoms like gas and bloating or more serious ones like diarrhea, constipation, or stomach pain.

Finding Sensitivities in Food

Food Diary: Keeping a thorough log of the foods you eat and the symptoms you experience might help you pinpoint possible causes.

Elimination Diet: This involves taking questionable items out of the diet for a short while before progressively adding them back in to see how the body responds.

Medical testing: Getting tests such as celiac disease screenings and lactose intolerance tests performed by medical specialists.

Handling Sensitive Foods

Dietary Adjustments: It's critical to alter the diet to exclude or restrict certain items when triggers have been discovered. Substitutes and alternatives may aid in keeping a diet in balance.

Examining Nutrition Labels: reading labels carefully and keeping an eye out for any hidden substances that can cause sensitivity reactions.

Having Sensitivities to Certain Foods

Meal Planning: Organizing meals and snacks that satisfy nutritional needs without triggering trigger foods.

Dining Out: When picking a restaurant, be sure to let them know about any dietary requirements you may have.

III Nutritional Sensitivities and Health

Promoting Gut Health: Eating a diet high in other gut-friendly foods, such high-fiber fruits and vegetables, probiotics, and prebiotics, helps promote general gut health in addition to avoiding trigger foods.

Supplements: For some illnesses, such as celiac disease, it may be required to take supplements such as lactase enzyme for lactose intolerance or vitamin and mineral supplements.

Handling Unintentional Exposure

Emergency Plan: Having a strategy in place in case of inadvertent consumption, which might include over-the-counter or prescription medicine to relieve symptoms.

Stress management is the awareness and control of the tension and worry that come with taking care of dietary sensitivity.

Establishing a Network of Support

Family and friends: Providing support and understanding in social situations by informing others in close proximity about the sensitivities.

Support Groups and Resources: Reaching out to others with like sensitivities to exchange experiences and advice.

Navigating Dining Out

For those who are committed to preserving intestinal health, eating out may be quite difficult, particularly for those who have particular dietary sensitivity or limits.

Getting Ready for a Restaurant Meal

Investigating Restaurants: Look for establishments that meet certain dietary requirements or provide gut-friendly alternatives before heading out to eat.

Examining Menus Ahead of Time: To determine whether products are appropriate for your dietary requirements, look at internet menus.

Interacting with the Restaurant: Don't be afraid to give them a call in advance to let them know about your dietary needs.

Making Knowledgeable Menu Selections

Identifying Safe Foods: Based on your unique requirements for gut health, know which foods are likely to be safe and which to avoid.

Posing Queries: Ask your waitress about the ingredients and processes used in the creation of menu items if you are unsure.

Simpler Dishes: Choose recipes with fewer ingredients since they are often simpler to evaluate and have a lower chance of include unidentified triggers.

Controlling Serving Sizes

Mindful Eating: Be mindful of portion proportions as consuming too much food might cause pain in the digestive tract. If you can, ask for a half-portion or consider sharing dishes.

Paying Attention to Your Body: Recognize when your body is hungry and full to prevent overindulging.

Techniques for Particular Dietary Requirements

Gluten-Free Dining: If you have a gluten sensitivity or celiac disease, look for restaurants that provide certified gluten-free menu items.

Low-FODMAP Options: If you're on a low-FODMAP diet, stick to basic proteins that are baked or grilled and stay away from high-FODMAP foods like onions and garlic.

Dairy-Free Options: Look out for hidden dairy in sauces and dressings and ask about dairy-free options.

Handling Differing Opinions

Concerns about Cross-Contamination: Crucial for those with severe food allergies or celiac disease. Verify that the employees of the restaurant are aware of the need to prevent cross-contamination.

Cooking Techniques: Find out how the restaurant prepares dishes free of allergens.

Gut Health and Alcohol

Reducing Alcohol Consumption: Red wine and other gut-friendly alternatives are good choices, but avoid alcohol altogether since it might irritate the stomach. Instead, go for non-alcoholic options.

Hydration: To keep hydrated, make sure you have plenty of water with any alcoholic drinks.

Managing Social Circumstances

Educating Companions: To assist your dining partners comprehend your food selections, let them know about your dietary requirements.

Savoring the Moment: Pay more attention to the fun and social aspects of dining out than the cuisine alone.

After-dinner observation

Symptom Monitoring: Keep an eye on how your body responds to meals you've eaten out to spot any foods that could not sit well with your stomach.

Emotional Eating and Gut Health
The widespread problem of eating out of emotion rather than hunger emotional eating can have a negative impact on intestinal health.

Recognizing Emotional Consumption

Definition and Triggers: Emotional eating refers to eating that is motivated by feelings other than actual hunger, such as stress, boredom, melancholy, or even enjoyment. Emotional anguish, indications from the environment, and certain psychiatric states are common triggers.

Effect on Digestive Health: Emotional eating on a regular basis may result in overindulgence, unhealthy eating choices, and digestive problems including bloating, pain, and gut flora imbalances.

Recognizing Emotional Eating Behaviors

Understanding Your Triggers: Being aware of the events, emotions, or periods of time that make you more prone to overindulge in food.

Food Diaries: You can spot emotional eating habits by keeping track of what you eat, when you consume it, and how you feel.

Techniques for Controlling Emotional Eating

Mindful Eating Practices: Savoring food, paying attention to hunger and fullness signals, and eating in the present.

Alternative Methods of Coping: establishing more constructive coping mechanisms for your emotions, such exercise, meditation, or hobbies.

Snacking Healthy: If you can't resist eating emotionally, go for gut-friendly snacks like fruits, veggies, or nuts.

Creating a Helpful Environment

Social Support: Accountability and motivation may be obtained by discussing your objectives with friends and family.

Dietary restrictions and emotional eating

Flexibility in Dieting: Giving yourself some leeway when it comes to your diet will help you feel less deprived, which helps prevent emotional eating.

Comfort Foods for a Gut Health: figuring out what meals are good for the stomach that would satiate emotional desires without making the gut worse.

Techniques for Relaxation and Stress Reduction

Relaxation Methods: Methods like progressive muscle relaxation, yoga, or deep breathing may help control the tension that often triggers emotional eating.

Frequent Exercise: Exercise helps control mood, hunger, and stress levels. It is also a powerful stress reliever.

Extended Behavior Modifications

Behavioral and Cognitive Techniques: Modifying the mental patterns that trigger emotional eating.

Understanding that altering one's eating habits is a gradual process that calls for patience and perseverance.

Staying Motivated and Consistent
A gut-healthy lifestyle takes consistent work and commitment. It may be difficult to maintain motivation and consistency, particularly in the face of daily pressures and temptations.

Having Reasonable Objectives

SMART Objectives: Establishing objectives that are Time-bound, Relevant, Measurable, Achievable, and Specific can help you monitor your progress and maintain motivation.

Small, Manageable adjustments: Gradual, small-scale adjustments are often more maintainable than abrupt ones.

Knowing the Reasons behind Your Objectives

Personal Health Benefits: Considering the advantages of a gut-healthy lifestyle for oneself, such as better digestion, more energy, and general wellbeing, may be quite motivating.

Pedagogical Approach: Ongoing education on gut health and its correlation with general well-being may bolster the significance of maintaining these practices.

Establishing a Network of Support

Community Support: Participating in online or in-person groups centered on gut health may provide accountability and motivation.

Family and Friends: Including your loved ones in your quest for gut health might provide extra encouragement and support.

Monitoring Development and Honoring Achievements

Monitoring Changes: You may show the beneficial effects of your efforts by monitoring changes in your energy levels, general well-being, and intestinal health.

Honoring Significant Occasions: No matter how little the accomplishment, acknowledging and appreciating it may increase drive.

Handling Obstacles

Acknowledging Variations: Realizing that obstacles are a typical aspect of any health journey and should not be used as an excuse to quit up.

Learning from Experiences: Determining the cause of the failure and devising a plan to avoid it in the future.

Including Fun and Variability

Dietary Variety: To make meals engaging and pleasurable, try out new, gut-friendly foods and cuisines.

Fun Physical Activities: To keep up a regular schedule, choose sports or activities you like.

Conscious and Perceptive Consuming

Listening to Your Body: Observing the impact of various meals on your digestive system and general well-being.

Slowing down, enjoying meals, and paying attention to feelings of hunger and fullness are examples of mindful eating practices.

Stress Reduction

Frequent Relaxation Practices: Make time each day for stress-relieving pursuits like yoga, meditation, or hobbies.

Good Coping Strategies: creating constructive coping mechanisms for stress that don't harm one's stomach.

12: Recipes for a Healthy Gut

Breakfast Ideas

Its common knowledge that breakfast is the most significant meal of the day, and this is particularly true in terms of gut health. Eating a gut-healthy breakfast may help your digestive system function better throughout the day.

1. Probiotic Yogurt Bowl
- Ingredients: Natural probiotic yogurt, mixed berries (blueberries, strawberries, raspberries), a sprinkle of chia seeds, and a drizzle of honey or maple syrup.
- Preparation: Layer the yogurt in a bowl, top with fresh berries, sprinkle with chia seeds, and drizzle with honey or maple syrup for a touch of sweetness.
- Benefits: Probiotic yogurt supports the gut microbiome, berries provide antioxidants, and chia seeds offer fiber.
2. Oatmeal with Prebiotic Toppings
- Ingredients: Rolled oats, almond milk, sliced bananas, chopped almonds, and a sprinkle of ground flaxseed.
- Preparation: Cook oats with almond milk, top with banana slices, almonds, and flaxseed.
- Benefits: Oats are a great source of soluble fiber, bananas provide prebiotics, and flaxseeds add omega-3 fatty acids.
3. Avocado Toast with Poached Egg
- Ingredients: Whole-grain bread, ripe avocado, poached egg, cherry tomatoes, and a pinch of salt and pepper.
- Preparation: Toast the bread, mash the avocado on top, add a poached egg, and garnish with cherry tomatoes, salt, and pepper.

- Benefits: Whole grains are rich in fiber, avocado provides healthy fats, and eggs offer high-quality protein.

4. Green Smoothie

- Ingredients: Spinach, kale, a green apple, a banana, Greek yogurt, and almond milk.
- Preparation: Blend all ingredients until smooth.
- Benefits: Leafy greens are nutrient-dense, the banana provides prebiotic fiber, and Greek yogurt adds probiotics.

5. Vegetable Omelette with Whole Grain Bread

- Ingredients: Eggs, spinach, bell peppers, onions, mushrooms, cheese, and whole-grain bread.
- Preparation: Sauté the vegetables, add beaten eggs, cook until set, and serve with a slice of whole-grain bread.
- Benefits: Eggs are a good protein source, vegetables add fiber and nutrients, and whole-grain bread is high in fiber.

6. Whole Grain Pancakes with Fruit Compote

- Ingredients: Whole-grain pancake mix, water or milk, and a compote made from mixed berries.
- Preparation: Prepare pancakes as directed and top with a homemade berry compote.
- Benefits: Whole grains are a good source of fiber, and berries provide essential vitamins and antioxidants.

7. Buckwheat Porridge with Mixed Nuts

- Ingredients: Buckwheat groats, almond milk, a mix of nuts (walnuts, almonds, cashews), cinnamon, and a touch of maple syrup.
- Preparation: Cook buckwheat in almond milk until tender. Stir in cinnamon and maple syrup. Top with a mix of chopped nuts.

- Benefits: Buckwheat is a good source of fiber and nutrients, while nuts add healthy fats and protein. Cinnamon can help regulate blood sugar levels.

8. Overnight Chia Pudding

- Ingredients: Chia seeds, almond milk, vanilla extract, and toppings like mixed nuts and berries.
- Preparation: Mix chia seeds with almond milk and vanilla, let sit overnight, and add toppings before serving.
- Benefits: Chia seeds are high in fiber and omega-3 fatty acids, nuts provide healthy fats, and berries offer antioxidants.

9. Quinoa Breakfast Bowl

- Ingredients: Cooked quinoa, sliced avocado, cherry tomatoes, a poached egg, and a sprinkle of pumpkin seeds.
- Preparation: Spoon warm quinoa into a bowl. Top with sliced avocado, cherry tomatoes, a poached egg, and sprinkle with pumpkin seeds.
- Benefits: Quinoa is a complete protein and rich in fiber, avocado provides healthy fats, tomatoes are rich in vitamins, and pumpkin seeds add a crunch with extra zinc and magnesium.

10. Savory Veggie Muffins

- Ingredients: Whole wheat flour, eggs, grated zucchini and carrots, diced bell peppers, a pinch of salt and pepper, and a bit of cheese.
- Preparation: Mix all ingredients and pour into muffin tins. Bake until set and golden.
- Benefits: Whole wheat flour provides fiber, vegetables add essential nutrients and fiber, and eggs offer protein.

11. Sweet Potato and Black Bean Breakfast Burrito

- Ingredients: Diced sweet potatoes, black beans, scrambled eggs, whole wheat tortillas, avocado, salsa, and a sprinkle of cheese.
- Preparation: Sauté sweet potatoes until tender, add black beans and scrambled eggs. Fill tortillas with the mixture, top with avocado and salsa, and sprinkle with cheese.
- Benefits: Sweet potatoes are high in fiber and vitamins, black beans add protein and fiber, and whole grains in tortillas support digestive health.

Lunch and Dinner Recipes

Keeping your gut healthy involves eating well at all times of the day, not just breakfast.

1. Grilled Salmon with Quinoa Salad

- Ingredients: Salmon fillets, quinoa, mixed greens (spinach, arugula), cherry tomatoes, cucumber, lemon juice, olive oil, salt, and pepper.
- Preparation: Grill the salmon. Cook quinoa as per instructions. Toss mixed greens, cherry tomatoes, and cucumber with cooked quinoa, dress with lemon juice and olive oil, season to taste. Serve with grilled salmon on top.
- Benefits: Salmon is rich in omega-3 fatty acids; quinoa provides fiber and protein; mixed greens offer a variety of nutrients and fiber.

2. Lentil Soup with Whole Grain Bread

- Ingredients: Lentils, carrots, celery, onions, garlic, vegetable broth, diced tomatoes, spinach, olive oil, herbs (thyme, bay leaf), and whole grain bread.

- Preparation: Sauté onions, garlic, carrots, and celery in olive oil. Add lentils, broth, tomatoes, and herbs. Simmer until lentils are tender, add spinach, and cook until wilted. Serve with whole grain bread.
- Benefits: Lentils are high in fiber and protein; vegetables add vitamins and antioxidants; whole grain bread is a good source of fiber.

3. Vegetable Stir-Fry with Brown Rice

- Ingredients: A variety of vegetables (broccoli, bell peppers, carrots, snap peas), tofu or chicken, brown rice, soy sauce, ginger, garlic, sesame oil.
- Preparation: Stir-fry vegetables and protein choice in sesame oil with ginger and garlic. Serve over cooked brown rice and drizzle with soy sauce.
- Benefits: Vegetables provide fiber and nutrients; brown rice is a whole grain rich in fiber; tofu or chicken adds protein.

4. Roasted Vegetable and Hummus Wraps

- Ingredients: Whole grain wraps, hummus, assorted vegetables (zucchini, bell peppers, onions, mushrooms), feta cheese, spinach or lettuce, olive oil, salt, and pepper.
- Preparation: Roast vegetables in olive oil, salt, and pepper. Spread hummus on wraps, add roasted vegetables, some feta, and a handful of spinach or lettuce. Roll up the wraps.
- Benefits: Hummus provides fiber and protein; vegetables are high in vitamins and antioxidants; whole grain wraps add fiber.

5. Mediterranean Chickpea Salad

- Ingredients: Chickpeas, cucumber, cherry tomatoes, red onion, olives, feta cheese, olive oil, lemon juice, parsley, salt, and pepper.

- Preparation: Mix chickpeas, cucumber, tomatoes, onion, and olives. Dress with olive oil and lemon juice, add feta and parsley, season to taste.
- Benefits: Chickpeas are a great source of fiber and protein; vegetables add a variety of nutrients; olive oil is rich in healthy fats.

6. Baked Sweet Potato with Black Bean Chili

- Ingredients: Sweet potatoes, black beans, tomatoes, onion, garlic, chili powder, cumin, olive oil, avocado, and Greek yogurt.
- Preparation: Bake sweet potatoes. Cook black beans with tomatoes, onion, garlic, and spices. Serve chili over sweet potatoes, topped with avocado and a dollop of Greek yogurt.
- Benefits: Sweet potatoes are high in fiber and vitamins; black beans provide fiber and protein; Greek yogurt adds probiotics.

7. Turmeric Chicken with Cauliflower Rice

- Ingredients: Chicken breasts, ground turmeric, garlic powder, olive oil, cauliflower (riced), assorted vegetables (e.g., peas, carrots), lemon juice, parsley.
- Preparation: Season chicken with turmeric, garlic powder, salt, and pepper. Cook in olive oil until done. Sauté riced cauliflower with vegetables, season with lemon juice and herbs. Serve chicken over cauliflower rice.
- Benefits: Turmeric is known for its anti-inflammatory properties; cauliflower is a low-carb, high-fiber alternative to rice; chicken provides lean protein.

8. Gut-Healing Bone Broth Soup

- Ingredients: Bone broth, diced vegetables (carrots, celery, onions), shredded chicken, kale or spinach, herbs (thyme, bay leaf), garlic, olive oil.

- Preparation: Sauté vegetables in olive oil with garlic. Add bone broth, cooked chicken, herbs, and simmer. Stir in leafy greens until wilted.
- Benefits: Bone broth provides collagen and amino acids for gut lining repair; vegetables and leafy greens offer fiber and nutrients.

9. Zucchini Noodles with Pesto and Cherry Tomatoes

- Ingredients: Zucchini (spiralized), cherry tomatoes, homemade pesto (basil, garlic, pine nuts, parmesan cheese, olive oil), lemon zest.
- Preparation: Sauté spiralized zucchini and cherry tomatoes in olive oil. Mix in homemade pesto and garnish with lemon zest.
- Benefits: Zucchini is a low-carb, high-fiber alternative to pasta; tomatoes are rich in antioxidants; pesto provides healthy fats and flavor.

10. Spicy Lentil Stew with Kale

- Ingredients: Lentils, kale, diced tomatoes, onion, garlic, vegetable broth, spices (cumin, paprika, cayenne pepper), olive oil.
- Preparation: Sauté onions and garlic in olive oil. Add lentils, broth, tomatoes, and spices. Simmer until lentils are tender. Stir in kale until wilted.
- Benefits: Lentils are a great source of plant-based protein and fiber; kale is nutrient-dense; spices add flavor and potential digestive benefits.

11. Grilled Tofu and Vegetable Skewers

- Ingredients: Firm tofu, bell peppers, onions, zucchini, mushrooms, tamari or soy sauce, ginger, garlic, olive oil.

- Preparation: Marinate tofu and vegetables in a mixture of tamari, ginger, and garlic. Thread onto skewers and grill until charred and cooked through.
- Benefits: Tofu is a good source of plant-based protein; a variety of vegetables ensures a broad intake of vitamins and fiber.

Snacks and Gut-Friendly Treats

When done correctly, snacks may be a beneficial component of a gut-friendly diet. Selecting foods that promote gut health is essential to preserving general well-being.

1. Roasted Chickpeas
- Ingredients: Canned chickpeas, olive oil, your choice of spices (e.g., cumin, paprika, garlic powder).
- Preparation: Drain and rinse chickpeas, toss with olive oil and spices, and roast in the oven until crispy.
- Benefits: Chickpeas are high in fiber and protein, making them an excellent snack for gut health.
2. Greek Yogurt with Honey and Walnuts
- Ingredients: Greek yogurt, a drizzle of honey, and a handful of walnuts.
- Preparation: Top Greek yogurt with a drizzle of honey and walnuts.
- Benefits: Greek yogurt is a great source of probiotics; honey provides natural sweetness; walnuts add healthy fats and texture.
3. Vegetable Sticks with Hummus
- Ingredients: Sliced raw vegetables (carrots, cucumbers, bell peppers), hummus.

- Preparation: Cut vegetables into sticks and serve with a bowl of hummus.
- Benefits: Vegetables are rich in vitamins and fiber; hummus provides protein and fiber.

4. Chia Seed Pudding

- Ingredients: Chia seeds, almond milk, a touch of maple syrup or honey, and a pinch of vanilla extract.
- Preparation: Mix chia seeds with almond milk, sweetener, and vanilla. Let it sit in the fridge to thicken. Top with fresh fruit before serving.
- Benefits: Chia seeds are rich in omega-3 fatty acids and fiber, which are excellent for gut health.

5. Homemade Granola Bars

- Ingredients: Oats, nuts, seeds, dried fruit, honey or maple syrup, and nut butter.
- Preparation: Mix ingredients, press into a baking dish, and bake until set. Cut into bars.
- Benefits: Oats are high in fiber; nuts and seeds provide healthy fats; dried fruits add natural sweetness.

6. Berry and Kefir Smoothie

- Ingredients: Mixed berries, kefir, a banana for sweetness, and a handful of spinach.
- Preparation: Blend all ingredients until smooth.
- Benefits: Berries are high in antioxidants; kefir is rich in probiotics; spinach adds fiber and nutrients.

7. Baked Apple Chips

- Ingredients: Thinly sliced apples, a sprinkle of cinnamon.
- Preparation: Arrange apple slices on a baking sheet, sprinkle with cinnamon, and bake until crispy.

- Benefits: Apples are a good source of fiber, particularly pectin, which is beneficial for gut health.

8. Dark Chocolate Squares

- Ingredients: High-quality dark chocolate (70% cocoa or higher).
- Preparation: Simply enjoy a square or two of dark chocolate.
- Benefits: Dark chocolate contains flavonoids that can have a prebiotic effect, feeding beneficial gut bacteria.

9. Nut and Seed Trail Mix

- Ingredients: A mix of almonds, walnuts, pumpkin seeds, sunflower seeds, dried cranberries or raisins, and a sprinkle of dark chocolate chips.
- Preparation: Combine all ingredients in a bowl and store in an airtight container for a convenient snack.
- Benefits: Nuts and seeds provide healthy fats, protein, and fiber, while dried fruits add natural sweetness and antioxidants.

10. Avocado Chocolate Mousse

- Ingredients: Ripe avocados, cocoa powder, maple syrup or honey, a pinch of salt, and vanilla extract.
- Preparation: Blend all ingredients until smooth for a creamy and healthy dessert.
- Benefits: Avocados are rich in monounsaturated fats and fiber; cocoa powder adds a dose of antioxidants.

Drinks and Smoothies

Gut health is largely dependent on hydration, and the things you drink may be just as significant as the things you consume.

1. Ginger Lemon Tea

- Ingredients: Fresh ginger root, lemon juice, honey, and hot water.

- Preparation: Grate ginger root into hot water, steep for several minutes, then strain. Add fresh lemon juice and honey to taste.
- Benefits: Ginger is known for its anti-inflammatory properties and can aid digestion; lemon is high in vitamin C; honey adds a soothing touch.

2. Green Detox Smoothie

- Ingredients: Spinach, kale, green apple, cucumber, celery, lemon juice, and a small piece of ginger.
- Preparation: Blend all ingredients until smooth, adding water to reach the desired consistency.
- Benefits: Leafy greens and green vegetables are rich in nutrients and fiber, aiding in digestion and detoxification.

3. Probiotic Berry Smoothie

- Ingredients: Mixed berries (blueberries, strawberries, raspberries), Greek yogurt or kefir, honey, and chia seeds.
- Preparation: Blend berries, yogurt or kefir, and honey until smooth. Stir in chia seeds and let sit for a few minutes before drinking.
- Benefits: Berries are high in antioxidants; yogurt or kefir provides probiotics; chia seeds add omega-3s and fiber.

4. Turmeric Golden Milk

- Ingredients: Almond milk, turmeric powder, cinnamon, ginger powder, black pepper, and honey.
- Preparation: Warm the almond milk, whisk in turmeric, cinnamon, ginger, and a pinch of black pepper. Sweeten with honey.
- Benefits: Turmeric and ginger are anti-inflammatory; cinnamon adds flavor and regulates blood sugar; black pepper increases turmeric absorption.

5. Watermelon Mint Cooler

- Ingredients: Fresh watermelon, mint leaves, lime juice, and ice cubes.
- Preparation: Blend watermelon with lime juice and mint leaves until smooth. Serve over ice.
- Benefits: Watermelon is hydrating and rich in lycopene, an antioxidant; mint can aid digestion.

6. Herbal Infusion

- Ingredients: Your choice of herbal tea (such as peppermint, chamomile, or fennel), hot water.
- Preparation: Steep the herbal tea in hot water according to package instructions.
- Benefits: Herbal teas can have various digestive health benefits, such as soothing the stomach and reducing bloating.

7. Cucumber Lemon Water

- Ingredients: Slices of cucumber, lemon, and fresh mint leaves, added to water.
- Preparation: Add cucumber, lemon slices, and mint to a pitcher of water and refrigerate for an hour or more.
- Benefits: This infused water is refreshing and hydrating, and cucumber adds a mild diuretic effect.

8. Beetroot and Carrot Juice

- Ingredients: Beetroot, carrot, apple, and a small piece of ginger.
- Preparation: Juice all ingredients, stir well and serve fresh.
- Benefits: Beetroot and carrots are high in fiber and nutrients that support gut health, while apple and ginger add flavor and digestive benefits.

9. Pineapple and Spinach Smoothie

- Ingredients: Fresh or frozen pineapple chunks, a handful of spinach, a banana, coconut water or almond milk, and a scoop of protein powder (optional).
- Preparation: Blend all ingredients until smooth. If needed, add more liquid to reach your preferred consistency.
- Benefits: Pineapple contains digestive enzymes called bromelain, spinach is rich in fiber and nutrients, and banana adds prebiotic fiber.

10. Kefir and Berry Smoothie

- Ingredients: Kefir, mixed frozen berries (such as blueberries, raspberries, and strawberries), a tablespoon of ground flaxseed, and a drizzle of honey or maple syrup for sweetness.
- Preparation: Blend the kefir, berries, and flaxseed until smooth. Sweeten to taste with honey or maple syrup.
- Benefits: Kefir is a fermented dairy product rich in probiotics; berries provide antioxidants; flaxseed adds omega-3 fatty acids and fiber.